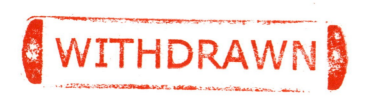

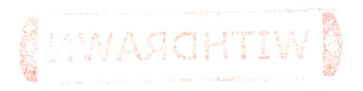

Visual Stress

OXFORD PSYCHOLOGY SERIES

Editors

Timothy Shallice	Nicholas J. Mackintosh
James L. McGaugh	Endel Tulving
Anne Treisman	Lawrence Weiskrantz

Visual Stress

Arnold J. Wilkins

MRC Applied Psychology Unit
Cambridge

OXFORD PSYCHOLOGY SERIES
NO. 24

Oxford New York Tokyo
OXFORD UNIVERSITY PRESS
1995

Oxford University Press, Walton Street, Oxford OX2 6DP

Oxford   New York
Athens   Auckland   Bangkok   Bombay
Calcutta   Cape Town   Dar es Salaam   Delhi
Florence   Hong Kong   Istanbul   Karachi
Kuala Lumpar   Madras   Madrid   Melbourne
Mexico City   Nairobi   Paris   Singapore
Taipei   Tokyo   Toronto
and associated companies in
Berlin Ibadan

Oxford is a trade mark of Oxford University Press

Published in the United States
by Oxford University Press Inc., New York

A catalogue record for this book is available from the British Library

Library of Congress Cataloging in Publication Data
(Data available on request)

ISBN 0 19 852174 X

Typeset by The Electronic Book Factory Ltd, Fife
Printed in Great Britain by
St. Edmundsbury Press, Bury St. Edmunds, Suffolk.

*Dedicated to all those
who suffer from visual discomfort,
especially Maria T.
—and to my wife, Liz,
children, Martha and Jonathan,
and parents, Leslie and Barbara.*

The eye is not satisfied with seeing
Ecclesiastes 1:8.

On the next page is a stressful pattern of stripes. **Do not look at this pattern if you have migraine or photosensitive epilepsy because it might provoke an attack.**

The pattern has a *square-wave luminance profile* (*duty cycle* 50%) with a *Michelson contrast* greater than 0.8. At a *viewing distance* of about 0.4m the radius is close to 14 deg. and the *spatial frequency* close to 3 cycle.deg^{-1}. Figure 3.1 shows that when patterns have these characteristics, anomalous perceptual effects, eye-strain, headaches, and seizures are possible.

Preface

In 1973 I was working as a post-doctoral research fellow in the Psychology Department at the Montreal Neurological Institute, with Brenda Milner. Frederick Andermann, a neurologist, referred one of his patients to the department and I was asked to see her. This book is dedicated to this patient, Maria T. She was a girl, then aged 14, who had seizures whenever she looked at striped patterns. The seizures consisted of a momentary loss of awareness, an *absence*, and they occurred *only* when she looked at striped patterns. Unfortunately for this little girl, stripes are everywhere in the modern urban environment: they are on clothes, furnishing fabrics, grills, gratings, and so forth. She was having an average of 22 absences an hour.

Pattern-sensitive epilepsy of this kind was then thought to be extremely rare. It was first described by Bickford in 1953, and since then only a few cases had been reported in the medical journals. By far the most intensive study had been by Chatrian *et al.* (1970), who had described four patients in detail. Hubel and Wiesel had recently made their momentous discovery of cells in the visual cortex of cats and monkeys that responded selectively to lines in certain orientations (see Hubel 1988). The parallels between the activity of these cells and of the cells that were triggering pattern-sensitive seizures were obvious.

Although Maria had been experiencing many absence seizures, they had lasted for only a few seconds and never developed into major motor convulsions. For this reason it seemed ethically acceptable to expose her to a variety of visual stimuli in the laboratory so as to investigate which stimuli did and which did not provoke a physiological response, in this case, a discharge of spike and slow waveforms on the electroencephalograph (EEG).

Most important from Maria's point of view was the finding that when one eye was covered, the sensitivity to patterns was greatly reduced. She was therefore given a pair of glasses with one lens frosted. Her seizures were monitored using the ambulatory EEG recording techniques, developed at the Montreal Neurological Institute by John Ives, that were then just becoming available. The EEG was recorded for four consecutive days. She wore the glasses on two of those days, and when she did so, the incidence of seizures was reduced from 22 per hour to 3 per hour.

Unfortunately the success in treating Maria was limited. She had many other handicaps in addition to her seizures, and the glasses did not prove to be a long-term success. The seizures were eventually controlled by *sodium valproate*, when the drug became available in North America. At the time, however, the short-term success in reducing seizures motivated me to continue studying pattern-sensitive epilepsy on my return to England to work at the MRC Applied Psychology Unit. I am grateful to the Medical Research Council and the director of the Applied Psychology Unit, Alan Baddeley, for giving me this opportunity.

I joined a team of people that had just begun an investigation of the mechanisms of a related form of reflex epilepsy: so-called *television epilepsy*, in which the viewing of television precipitates seizures. The team included Colin Binnie, then in charge of Clinical Neurophysiology at St Bartholomew's Hospital, and Colleen Darby, then Chief Physiological Measurement Technician at Runwell Hospital. We began a study together with Siggy Stefansson which was to show that pattern-sensitivity was far more prevalent than had been thought, and that it was responsible for many of the problems associated with television. These findings are described in Chapters 2 and 7. The discovery that pattern sensitivity was not rare but could be demonstrated in many patients if the appropriate pattern was used, led to a series of detailed studies of the stimulus characteristics. The effects of the pattern shape, size, contrast, and brightness were investigated, and these are described in Chapter 2.

We were eventually able to design visual stimuli that were maximally likely to induce the EEG abnormalities associated with epilepsy and these stimuli are now used as a diagnostic tool. Patients' relatives would often comment: 'Oh, I could not look at *that* for long – it would give me a headache.' It soon became apparent that we had produced a very uncomfortable stimulus, not necessarily for the patients with epilepsy – they rarely suffered discomfort – but for people with other complaints.

The complaints of discomfort from people without epilepsy were reminiscent of the complaints of eye-strain that had been associated with the recent introduction of video displays for use with computers. I wondered whether the flicker from computer screens was one of the causes of the complaints because many photosensitive patients suffered seizures when they were close to television screens. I began by checking this in a rather roundabout way. I asked normal observers to rate the pleasantness of patterns of stripes with different spacing. Not only were the stripes that provoked seizures rated as being the most unpleasant, many observers subsequently complained of headaches and dizziness. They reported anomalous visual effects: illusions of colour, shape, and motion, and some observers were far more susceptible to these illusions than others. It was a short step to find out whether the observers who reported many illusions were those who were generally more susceptible to headaches, and this indeed turned out to be the case. Moreover, the stimuli most likely to provoke discomfort and illusions were almost exactly the same as those most likely to provoke seizures. These findings are described in Chapter 3.

It took me some time to realize that text could be considered as a pattern of stripes, and that at least some of the eye-strain associated with reading could be attributed to this pattern. At first I thought that the stripes were too broken up and of too low a contrast, but after listening to patients describing their symptoms I thought it would be worthwhile doing some measurements. These measurements seemed to confirm that the lines of text could be considered to be stripes. Two strands of evidence finally convinced me: (1) an unbiased observer described illusions from text identical to those from stripes; (2) covering the lines above and below those being read (removing the stripes) reduced seizures and headaches. Eventually Roger Watt and I filtered samples of text having different typographic characteristics and showed how these characteristics affected the striped properties.

Illusions and complaints of discomfort are subjective and difficult to measure. I tried to find objective indices of visual function that might be associated with the discomfort, and an obvious place to start was with eye movements. Two experts in the field, John Findlay and Roger Carpenter, kindly helped me obtain some pilot data which suggested that such an approach might be worthwhile. They helped set up the necessary recording equipment based on a personal computer that IBM donated and an analogue – digital converter made by Mike Gartrell in the IBM laboratories at Hursley.

The relationships between eye movements and the occurrence of illusions in patterns proved to be difficult to measure, partly because the movements that occur when the eyes are looking at something are extremely small. The effects of flicker from visual displays were more substantial. Large rapid eye movements (saccades) are often followed by smaller corrective movements that serve to bring the centre of gaze closer to the desired point in space. I found that the number of these corrective movements was increased on a video display, owing to the flicker. Further experiments showed that this increase may occur because the flicker interferes with the mechanisms that prevent our seeing the visual world during the eye movement itself. These experiments are described in Chapters 6 and 7.

Fluorescent lighting pulsates in brightness 100 times per second (120 in America). It had been in use for three decades, but a steady trickle of complaints of associated headaches and eye-strain still persisted. The pulsation from fluorescent lighting is too rapid to see, and strictly speaking, cannot therefore be called 'flicker'. Nevertheless nerve cells in the eyes and brain respond to each pulsation. Having found a small effect of the pulsation on the control of eye movements, I thought it would be worthwhile to see whether the pulsation was also responsible for headaches. A new form of fluorescent lighting had just become commercially available. It used electronic circuitry to remove most of the 100-per-second pulsation. With the help of Anthony Slater at the Building Research Establishment and Lou Bedocs of Thorn Lighting I was able to set up a headache and eye-strain survey in a large office block, changing the form of lighting during the course of the survey. Much to my surprise, the office workers reported only half the usual number of headaches under the new lighting. These findings are described in Chapter 6.

The new form of lighting was relatively expensive to install (although much cheaper to run) so I wondered how the effects of the pulsation from conventional lamps could be reduced in other ways. I measured the pulsation from a wide variety of lamps and found that for the most common types of lamp the pulsation was greatest at the blue end of the spectrum. Together with Peter Wilkinson, then at Cambridge Optical Group, I designed a spectacle tint to reduce the pulsation. The tint has a rosy-brown appearance. These spectacles were very similar to some of those designed by Helen Irlen for use by people with dyslexia.

I had already come across reports of Helen Irlen's work in the media. She uses coloured glasses to treat a condition she has called 'scotopic sensitivity syndrome' from which many people with dyslexia are said to suffer. I had been intrigued by the similarity between the symptoms of this syndrome and the distortions seen in patterns of stripes. Together with Catherine Neary, a colleague with a background in optometry (who was supported by the Health and Safety Executive), I examined a group of patients who had been to the Irlen Institute and had received specially tinted spectacles. The reports of the patients convinced me that the treatment could be very beneficial, although the objective results of the optometric examination were certainly insufficient to convince clinical colleagues. I designed a simple apparatus for examining the perceptual effects of colour in a systematic way. Bob Edwards helped me build it. This apparatus turned out to provide a rapid and precise technique for assessing ophthalmic tints. A set of tints was developed with advice from R. W. G. Hunt, and is now part of a system for ophthalmic tinting that is commercially available and patented by the MRC. A large team including Bruce Evans and Jenny Brown helped me to run a double-blind trial to evaluate the system. The trial demonstrated that the benefits people reported were more than could be attributed to placebo. The tinting system and its evaluation are described in Chapter 9.

I offer this autobiographical introduction so that readers can get an idea of how things actually came about, rather than how, with hindsight, they should have come about. The latter form of introduction is more commonly found in scientific texts and such an introduction is offered in Chapter 1!

I am grateful to my colleagues and friends in Cambridge, particularly Ian Nimmo-Smith who has offered help with statistics on many joint projects,

Roger Watt for his ideas on images and Kalvis Jansons for criticism. I thank Horace Barlow and Simon Laughlin who gave me some of the ideas in Chapter 10. Fergus Campbell and John Robson offered their advice and support over many years, and kindly looked through a draft of the manuscript. The book owes much to the pioneering work of these two scientists, and it is offered in memory of Fergus Campbell. Their comments, and those of Edward Chronicle, Bruce Evans, Peter Gloor, Chris Kennard, Anne Maclachlan, and James Tresilian, are much appreciated. Brenda Milner taught me about science and the brain: I hope I learned a little. My family, Elizabeth, Martha, and Jonathan, helped me write English, so they certainly deserve a mention, as indeed do so many others . . .

Cambridge   A.J.W.
April 1994

Contents

1 Introduction

A general and unified theory of visual discomfort is outlined in Chapters 2–4 and is then applied to a variety of everyday problems, such as eye-strain from reading (Chapter 5), from lighting (Chapter 6), from television and visual display terminals (Chapter 7), and more generally from design (Chapter 8). The role of colour in therapy is reviewed in Chapters 9 and 10, and the Appendix gives a summary of techniques for preventing discomfort.

Some things are unpleasant to look at by virtue of what they represent, and others because of their intrinsic physical properties. A picture of a traffic accident is one example of a visual stimulus that is unpleasant because of the pain and suffering that it signifies and the emotion that it engenders. Unpleasant though such scenes undoubtedly are, they do not leave the eyes feeling tired and they do not cause a sensation 'like to a knife being driven through the eye'. Visual stimuli that have these unpleasant effects do exist, and the effects occur because of the physical properties of the stimuli, quite independently of any semantic association. This book attempts to explain the mechanisms of such 'eye-strain'.

Eye-strain is a term that is used colloquially to refer to discomfort or pain in or around the eyes, and such discomfort is very common. Although there are many possible causes for pain with this localization, the causes are easy to recognize only when the pain is the result of an obvious disorder of the eye. For example, an ulcer on the front of the eye can be intensely painful. This is not a common cause for pain in the eye, and for the most part, the pain of eye-strain remains poorly understood. This book offers a theory of visual discomfort that seeks to interpret the discomfort in terms of a neurological response to excessive visual processing. Couched in a dictum, the message of this book is simply: 'Eye-strain is brain-strain', or, more accurately, 'some eye-strain is brain-strain'. There are undoubtedly many causes of pain in and around the eyes that are little to do with the brain, and they are not the concern of this book. I hope that optometrists do not find this too great an omission.

The theory is pieced together from a large number of fragmentary items of evidence. Considered individually, each item might be taken to be a part of a different picture, but when taken together the various fragments seem to fit together. They are rather like the pieces of a wet cardboard jigsaw puzzle! Although each piece of evidence is soft and malleable, it fits with the other pieces to form a cohesive interlocking structure. The picture is still only partially complete and remains somewhat blurred, but it has now 'dried out' sufficiently to be worth describing.

Visual stimulation can give rise to a variety of adverse effects, including anomalous perceptual phenomena, distortions of various kinds, discomfort, nausea, dizziness, aches and pains in and around the eyes, headaches, and even epileptic seizures. The theory offered in this book is unified and general: it is intended to apply to all these adverse consequences of visual stimulation, and to explain why similar visual stimuli can be responsible for such effects. Chapter 2 is devoted to a description of the stimuli responsible for epileptic seizures, and the physiological mechanisms whereby the seizures are induced. In Chapter 3 it is shown that the stimuli capable of inducing seizures in patients with photosensitive epilepsy are the same stimuli that evoke in others perceptual distortion, feelings of discomfort, eye-strain, and headaches. The perceptual distortion is associated with the eye-strain and headaches in a variety of ways. In Chapter 4 these threads are drawn together. It is shown that the visual stimuli responsible for adverse effects are those:

(1) to which the visual system is most sensitive;

(2) that interfere with the perception of other stimuli;

(3) that give rise to a large electrical and vascular response in the brain.

Once the theory has been developed in Chapters 2–4, it is applied to everyday problems. Chapter 5 deals with eye-strain from reading, and is devoted to the effects of spatially confusing patterns in textual material. In Chapter 6 some of the detrimental effects of the rapid pulsation of light are summarized. Electronic displays are described in the next chapter, and in this chapter the pulsation of light and the spatial structure of text are considered together, in relation to complaints of visual discomfort from visual display terminals. The consequences for design are briefly considered in Chapter 8, with case histories of poor design as examples.

In Chapter 9 there follows a description of a new system for precision tinting, and the therapeutic promise that it holds. Theoretical speculations concerning the role of colour in the reduction of visual discomfort are offered in Chapter 10, and the Appendix provides an overview of techniques for avoiding discomfort, for the benefit of sufferers.

2 Photosensitive epilepsy

2.1 Introduction

About 4 per cent of patients with epilepsy are liable to visually induced seizures. The visual stimulation responsible includes both flickering light and stationary steadily illuminated patterns, usually of stripes. The seizures can start in the visual cortex of one cerebral hemisphere or both hemispheres independently. The seizures occur when normal physiological excitation involves more than a critical cortical area, particularly when the excitation is rhythmic.

2.1.1 The epilepsies: cause and localization

Epilepsy is defined as a liability to recurrent seizures. Seizures arise from an abnormal discharge of neurones in the brain. The cause is often unknown, in which case the epilepsy is said to be *idiopathic*. Sometimes a structural brain lesion may be observable (in which case the epilepsy is *symptomatic*); or it may be reasonable to assume that there is such a lesion on the basis of clinical signs (in which case the epilepsy is *cryptogenic*). The epilepsy is classified not only on the basis of its cause, but also its localization within the brain. The epilepsy may be *generalized* involving all brain regions, or *partial*, confined to a specific region of the brain, usually within the temporal or frontal lobes, structures that are relatively easily damaged by lack of oxygen.

Four diagnostic categories are based on the above nomenclature: idiopathic generalized epilepsy, symptomatic generalized epilepsy, idiopathic partial epilepsy, and symptomatic partial epilepsy. In each of the diagnostic categories the seizures may take a variety of forms, ranging from the bilateral rhythmic tonic clonic movements of a generalized major motor seizure to a momentary lapse of full awareness, which can sometimes be so fleeting as to pass unnoticed, both by patients and people around them. The classification of epileptic seizures is therefore complex and controversial. For the present it is sufficient to note that patients often suffer more than one type of seizure, and that the behavioural manifestations of a seizure may be extremely subtle.

In about 4 per cent of patients with epilepsy, seizures may be provoked by visual stimulation, and in many of these patients the seizures occur *only* in response to visual stimulation. (181 of the 454 photosensitive patients reported by Jeavons and Harding (1975, p. 32) had seizures only in response

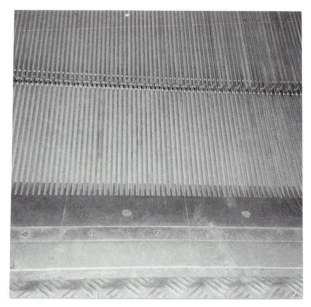

Fig. 2.1 The pattern of stripes formed by the metal stair tread of an escalator. The pattern has characteristics that are similar to those for which seizures are most likely.

to flicker.) Usually the seizures are provoked by flickering light, as from discotheque stroboscopes and television, or when sunlight is interrupted by road-side trees, or reflected from waves on the surface of a lake. Occasionally geometric patterns can also be responsible: one pattern that can provoke seizures is provided by the stripes on the metal stair tread of certain escalators (see Fig. 2.1).

Light sensitivity is most common in idiopathic generalized epilepsy, although all categories of epilepsy may be photosensitive. Any type of seizure may be triggered by light stimulation.

2.1.2 The clinical EEG examination in photosensitive epilepsy

In patients with epilepsy the electrical activity of the brain can be abnormal between seizures as well as during them. For this reason, patients are usually examined with the help of the *electroencephalograph* (EEG). The minute voltages emanating from the brain are recorded using electrodes (usually silver discs with a coating of silver chloride) held against the scalp. The differences in electrical potential between pairs of electrodes or between each electrode and some combination of other electrodes are amplified electronically. The amplified signals are recorded (usually on moving paper) so as to show the moment-to-moment fluctuations in voltage that form the *electroencephalogram*. The fluctuations are due, in part, to the activity of neurones in the brain beneath. The relatively large pyramidal neurones are thought to be mainly responsible. These are oriented perpendicularly to the surface of the brain and their collective activity provides a varying electrical field. The orientation of this field with respect to the electrodes determines where on the surface of the scalp the neural activity may most easily be recorded. The neurones in the *striate cortex* (one of the visual areas of the brain) are hidden in the gap between the cerebral hemispheres at the back of the head (the *calcarine fissure*). The electrical field from these neurones is therefore oriented in such a way that the activity of neurones in the right hemisphere is recorded on the left side of the scalp (Blumhardt *et al.* 1978): there is an anomalous lateralization of activity. Other visual structures are not hidden in the calcarine fissure and their activity is recorded where you might expect it: on the same side of the head as that on which the neural activity occurs.

Figure 2.2 shows an EEG tracing from a patient with epilepsy. The scale shows the calibration and the inset maps the position of the electrodes on the scalp and the combinations of electrodes between which the voltage has been measured. The fluctuations in voltage may be likened to the vibrations that you can feel on the outer casing of a piano when several notes are played simultaneously. Many different frequencies (or 'notes') are present in the voltage fluctuations, and not all arise from brain activity. There is electrical contamination from muscle activity (mainly high frequency) and from changes in electrode impedance (mainly low frequency). The contamination can be reduced by filtering the signal so that only frequencies between about 3 and 50 per second are displayed.

The record in Fig. 2.2 is entirely normal until the patient looks at a flickering light. Each flash of the light is shown on the bottom channel. After a few flashes the tracing shows spikes and large slow waves that were not previously present. The waveforms comprise one example of a so-called *photoconvulsive response*[1] (Bickford *et al.* 1953), a misnomer because the patient does not convulse: indeed there may be no outward clinical signs and sometimes no awareness of any abnormal sensation on the part of the patient.

---

[1] This term is reserved for a discharge with the following characterstics: (1) there are regular or irregular single or multiple spikes interspersed with slow waves; (2) the time at which each spike occurs is independent of the times at which the flashes occur, i.e. the spikes are not phase-locked to the flashes; (3) the spikes and slow waves have a frequency between 2.5 and 3 per second; (4) the discharge is fairly symmetrical either side of the head; and (5) it is seen over all head regions (although often maximal on channels towards the front of the head).

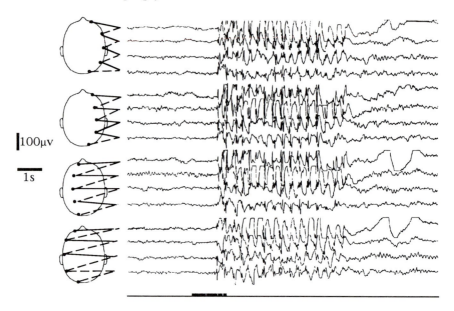

Fig. 2.2 An EEG recording from a 12 year old boy with photosensitive epilepsy. The lines are drawn by pens that trace the difference in electrical potential between pairs of electrodes on the scalp, positioned as shown in the diagram. The bottom channel records flashes of intermittent light.

The response shown in Fig. 2.2 outlasts the flashes. Such a response has considerable diagnostic significance because when it occurs the chances are about 90 per cent that the patient has previously suffered some form of epileptic seizure, occurring either spontaneously or during provocative visual stimulation (Reilly and Peters 1973)[2]. The few people who exhibit a photoconvulsive response but do not have a history of seizures are usually close relatives of people with epilepsy (Jeavons and Harding 1975, p. 43 *et seq.*).

The fact that intermittent light can elicit an EEG response that is strongly associated with epilepsy is one of the reasons why clinical EEG examinations routinely include stimulation with intermittent light. The intermittent light is usually provided by a xenon gas discharge lamp that presents a train of very intense but very brief flashes. (The apparent brightness is similar to that of a television displaying a white scene.) The flashes are turned off as soon as a photoconvulsive response appears, to prevent the discharge developing into

---

[2] The light is usually turned off immediately a photoconvulsive response occurs, and whether or not the discharge outlasts the flashes obviously depends to some extent on the speed with which this action is taken.

a seizure. In this way it is possible to assess epileptic photosensitivity with only a very small risk of seizures.

Many patients who show a photoconvulsive response to intermittent light also show a response to certain patterns, even when the patterns are steadily illuminated. If the patterns have the appropriate spatial characteristics, about half the patients show pattern-sensitivity (Darby *et al.* 1980). The proportion increases to 70 per cent if the patterns vibrate with the appropriate displacement and velocity.

The *paroxysmal* (i.e. short-lived) EEG response to patterns is usually less marked than that to intermittent light: it has a lower voltage, is manifest on fewer electrodes, and may have fewer types of waveforms. In other words, a pattern stimulus is usually less *epileptogenic*. The paroxysmal response from a pattern stimulus nevertheless shares the *epileptiform* spikes, sharp, or slow waves characteristically associated with epilepsy.

2.2 The visual stimulation that causes seizures

The paroxysmal epileptiform EEG response, like seizures, is probabilistic: sometimes it occurs, and sometimes it does not. The probability of the response can be estimated by repeatedly presenting the pattern and noting the proportion of presentations on which the epileptiform activity occurs. It turns out that the probability depends on the characteristics of the visual stimulus in a predictable way.

2.2.1 Flicker

The epileptogenic properties of a flickering light might be expected to depend on the size of the retinal image of the source, its time-averaged luminance, the *modulation* of the light (i.e. the proportionate change in luminance with each flash), the frequency of the modulation, the colour of the light (or more precisely, its *spectral power distribution*), and the part of the retina receiving stimulation. Far more is known about the effects of frequency than any other variable.

Frequency
Jeavons and Harding (1975) studied a sample of 170 photosensitive patients. The proportion of the sample showing a photoconvulsive response is shown in Fig. 2.3 (solid line) as a function of flash frequency. About half the patients were sensitive at frequencies of 50 Hz, although nearly all were sensitive when the frequency was close to 20 Hz. These are group data. Individual patients do not always show maximum sensitivity at 20 Hz. The sensitivity for one such individual is shown in Fig. 2.3 (broken line).

Colour

There are four types of photoreceptors in the eye: the *rods* (active mainly at twilight) and three categories of *cones* (active at higher luminance levels and sensitive mainly to short-, medium-, or long-wavelength light). The sensation of colour is derived from the output of the cones by complex neural computation. There have been many investigations of the effects of coloured light on the photoconvulsive response. Early studies did not control for the change in luminance associated with the use of a coloured filter. Jeavons and Harding (1975) reviewed the literature, including studies of their own in which a xenon lamp was covered with a coloured filter. They came to the conclusion that if allowance is made for luminance, all colours of light are almost equally epileptogenic. Takahashi and Tsukahara (1976), however, reported that red light is more epileptogenic than white. Binnie *et al.* (1984) attempted to reconcile these findings, arguing that a deep red colour may avoid the inhibitory interactions between receptor classes. Whilst this is possible, the inconsistency in the literature may also have a simpler interpretation. As we will see in Chapter 9, there are large differences between individuals in the response to colour. Although individual patients may show greater susceptibility to certain colours than to others (Newmark and Penry 1979, p. 131), the differences between individuals mean that the population as a whole may show little consistency.

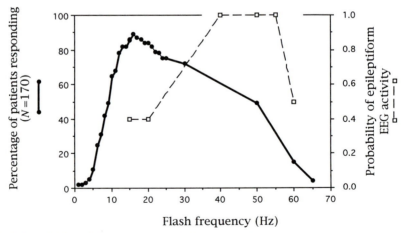

Fig. 2.3 *Solid line*: The proportion of photosensitive patients showing a photocon-vulsive EEG response to intermittent light, expressed as a function of flash frequency (after Jeavons and Harding 1975). *Broken line*: The probability of epileptiform EEG activity in a single patient, estimated by repeated randomized trails (after Wilkins *et al.* 1980).

Few studies have investigated the therapeutic effects of wearing coloured spectacles. Newmark and Penry (1979) reviewed reports of successful treatment in single cases, although there was no consistency as to choice of colour. The therapeutic effects of coloured spectacles are considered in detail in Chapter 9.

Other characteristics

Many other characteristics of flickering light undoubtedly contribute to its epileptogenic effects, but their contribution is not well described. We know that the light does not have to appear in brief flashes: it can be epileptogenic if it alternates bright and dim for equal periods of time, varying gradually (as a sine-wave) or abruptly (as a square-wave). The luminance (averaged over time) can be as low as 20 cd m^{-2}, the modulation as low as 40 per cent and the variation still be sufficient to provoke epileptiform EEG activity in some photosensitive patients.

Stimulation at the centre of gaze is far more effective than stimulation in the periphery of the visual field, despite the fact that flicker is often most visible 'out of the corner of the eye' (Jeavons and Harding 1975). As we will see in Section 2.3 this is because less of the cortex is devoted to the analysis of the periphery of vision.

The duration of stimulation is undoubtedly very important: brief two-second bursts of intermittent light are used in the routine EEG recording because they can provoke epileptiform EEG activity that does not progress to seizures. The longer the stimulation the greater the chances of a seizure, although, for obvious reasons, the effects of duration have not been studied.

2.2.2 Pattern

When Stefansson *et al.* (1977) discovered that many photosensitive patients are sensitive to patterns as well as to flicker, it seemed important to try to ascertain the nature of the patterns responsible. Wilkins *et al.* (1975, 1979a, 1980, 1981) studied the stimulus characteristics using the following simple technique. Patterns printed on card were attached to a wand and held against a screen, see Fig. 2.4. The screen was diffusely lit with steady white light and reflected the same amount of light as the patterns. The patterns bore a central *fixation point* at which the patient was instructed to gaze. Patterns were generally presented for 10 s unless epileptiform activity occurred, when they were removed immediately. No major motor seizures were induced using this technique, and the patients rarely experienced any unpleasant sensation. The testing was stopped if the patient wished, or if they became tired. The epileptogenic effects of patterns could be studied using

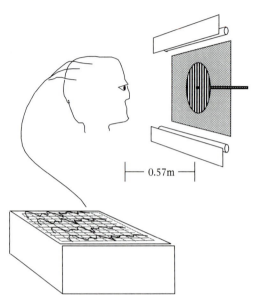

0.57m

Fig. 2.4 The techniques for pattern testing. The patient sat at a distance of 0.57 m from a grey screen diffusely lit by high-frequency white fluorescent lamps above and below. Patterns, printed on card, were attached to a wand and held against the screen by the examiner. The EEG was recorded using conventional techniques.

this technique without prolonged exposure to patterns and with a minimum of discomfort or risk.

The patterns most likely to provoke epileptiform EEG activity are striped, with long line contours. Figure 2.5 shows the data from a single patient who observed patterns of checks in which the checks were stretched along one dimension (Wilkins *et al.* 1975, 1979a). The longer the length of the checks, the greater the probability of epileptiform EEG activity, and the more the pattern approximated a grating pattern.

Parameters of gratings

Gratings are commonly used in vision research because they are some of the simplest patterns: they vary in one dimension only. If a light meter is moved along that dimension, the luminance varies cyclically according to a particular profile. This *luminance profile* can vary with respect to its mean, and the proportion that it varies about the mean (known as the *contrast*). In Figs 2.6(a)–(c), l_2 and l_1 are the maximum and minimum luminances respectively. The mean luminance is $[x.l_2+(s-x).l_1]/s$ which, in the symmetrical profiles shown in Fig. 2.6(b) and (c) reduces to $(l_2+l_1)/2$. The contrast is expressed as the *Michelson* fraction: $(l_2-l_1)/(l_2+l_1)$.

The angle one cycle subtends at the eye (α in Fig. 2.6(d)) is a measure of the size of the image that the bars of the pattern cast on the *retina* of light-sensitive cells at the back of the eye. When describing repetitive patterns, it is conventional to refer to the reciprocal of this angle as *spatial frequency*. Thus the spatial frequency of a pattern is the number of pattern cycles in one degree subtended at the eye, $1/\alpha$.

In the profile illustrated in Fig. 2.6(a) the luminance varies according to a *rectangular-wave*: the luminance shifts abruptly between two values. The bars therefore have sharp edges. The pattern can vary with respect to the proportion of one cycle for which the luminance is high. This is known as the *duty cycle*, and in Fig. 2.6(a) the duty cycle is x/s (=25 per cent). In Fig. 2.6(b), the rectangular wave is a *square-wave* in which the luminance is

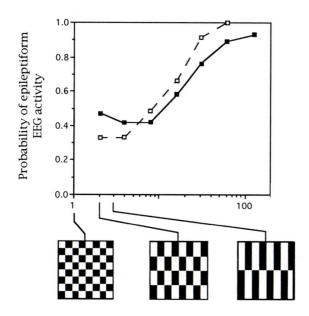

Length/width ratio of line segments

Fig. 2.5 The probability of epileptiform EEG activity in response to chequered patterns. The checks have been stretched as shown, and the probability is expressed as a function of the length/width ratio of the checks. The data are from a single patient tested in two sessions. The width of the checks subtended 6 min of arc in one session (continuous line) and 12 min in the other (broken line). The pattern was square in outline, and its side subtended 12.5 deg. The luminance contrast of the checks was 9×10^{-1} and the mean luminance about 3×10^{-1} cd m^{-2}. (After Wilkins *et al.* 1979*a*.) The patterns below the *x*-axis illustrate the change in length/width ratio schematically.

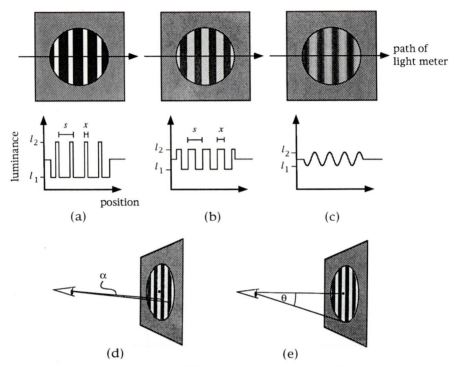

Fig. 2.6 (a) – (c) Patterns with different luminance profiles. The horizontal arrow shows the path across the pattern traced by a light meter, and the graphs beneath show the luminance profile measured by the meter. The luminance varies between l_2 and l_1, as shown. The luminance contrast of the pattern is given by the Michelson ratio, $(l_2 - l_1/(l_2 + l_1)$. In (b) the luminance profile is a square wave, and in (c) a sine wave. The duty cycle is x/s. In (d) one cycle of the pattern subtends the angle α at the eye, and the spatial frequency of the pattern is therefore $1/\alpha$ cycle deg^{-1}. (e) The pattern is circular in outline with an angular radius of Θ.

alternately high and low for the same distance. The duty cycle of the grating in Fig. 2.6(b) is therefore $x/s=50$ per cent.

The gratings commonly used in vision research have a different profile in which luminance varies as a sine-wave, and the bars therefore have indistinct edges, see Fig. 2.6(c). The reason for this choice is to be found in the application of Fourier analysis to spatial vision begun by Campbell and Robson (1968). Fourier's theorem states that any function can be made by adding sine-waves together. This is illustrated in Fig. 2.7. A square-wave, for example, can be made by adding an infinite number of sine-waves together, beginning with a sine-wave that has a spatial frequency the same as that of the square-wave, known as the *fundamental*, see Fig. 2.7(a). To this fundamental are added a succession of sine-waves with higher spatial frequencies (*harmonics*). In the case of a square-wave, the frequency, *amplitude*, and *phase* of the harmonics bear a simple relationship to those of the fundamental. The amplitude refers to the vertical distance between peaks, and the phase to the horizontal position. The amplitude of the *even harmonics* (those with spatial frequencies 2, 4, ... times that of the fundamental) is zero. The *third harmonic* (with a spatial frequency three times that of the fundamental) has an amplitude one third that of the fundamental and a phase such that the troughs occur at the same place as the peaks of the fundamental. Figure 2.7(b) shows the third harmonic and Fig. 2.7(c) shows the waveform that results when the third harmonic is added to the fundamental. The fifth harmonic (Fig. 2.7(e)) has a phase such that the peaks add to those of the fundamental. When all the harmonics have been added, the end result is a square-wave with an amplitude 0.785 ($\pi/4$) times that of the fundamental.

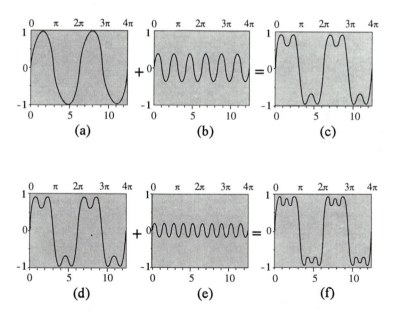

Fig. 2.7 Fourier components of a square-wave. (a) The fundamental. (b) The third harmonic. When the fundamental and the third harmonic are added, as in (c) and, similarly, (d), the waveform begins to resemble a square-wave. When the fifth harmonic, shown in (e) is added, the curve in (f) results, which has a greater resemblance to a square-wave. If the addition of odd harmonics is continued to infinity a square-wave results. The even harmonics of a square-wave are zero.

Response to complex gratings

Soso *et al.* (1980*a*, *b*) examined a single patient with pattern-sensitive epilepsy, comparing the amount of epileptiform EEG activity in response to various sine-wave gratings with that in response to a complex grating. The complex grating had a profile similar to Fig. 2.7(c). It was formed by adding two sinusoidal gratings together, one with a contrast of 15 per cent and a spatial frequency of 5 cycle deg^{-1} and the other with a contrast of 5 per cent and a spatial frequency of 15 cycle deg^{-1}. Epileptiform activity occurred in response to sinusoidal gratings with spatial frequencies in the range 1–9 cycle deg^{-1} but was most prevalent when the spatial frequency was 5 cycle deg^{-1}. The complex grating induced even more epileptiform activity than the 5 cycle deg^{-1} grating. In other words, the sharper the edges of the bars in a pattern, the greater the activity. The complex grating presumably stimulated more visual neurones, those sensitive to the fundamental and those sensitive to the higher harmonics. The results suggest that the greater the physiological excitation induced by the pattern, the greater its epileptogenic effects.

The third harmonic of the grating in Fig. 2.7(c) has been added to approximate a square-wave grating. If the phase of the harmonic is shifted so that the peaks of the curves add rather than subtract, the resulting waveform approximates a triangle wave. In a second study Soso *et al.* (1980*a*) found that gratings with such a luminance profile had an epileptogenic effect similar to that when the components approximated a square-wave: in other words it was not the sharp edges that rendered the grating epileptogenic, but the amplitude of the components; the phase of the components did not appear to matter. The total energy in the pattern seemed to be the relevant variable.

When a checkerboard is subjected to two-dimensional Fourier analysis, most of the contrast energy is in the diagonals. The diagonals form two crossing 'striped' patterns, as it were, and the contrast energy in the pattern is divided between these diagonal orientations. When the checks are stretched, as in Fig. 2.5, the energy shifts from the diagonals and eventually all the energy is in one orientation, that of the main axis along which contrast varies, i.e. at right-angles to the stripes. The increase in epileptiform activity with the length of the stripes shown in Fig. 2.5 can therefore be interpreted as resulting from the concentration of energy within one orientation. This interpretation is supported by the finding of Wilkins *et al.* (1979*a*). In their study two orthogonal gratings were added optically, giving a plaid pattern similar to that in Fig. 2.8(c). The energy in the resulting pattern was confined to the vertical and the horizontal orientations. When one of the gratings was replaced by a diffuse uniform field with the same space-averaged luminance, a single lower contrast grating remained, shown in Fig. 2.8(f). Although the luminance contrast in this grating was less than that in the figure in Fig. 2.8(c), the epileptogenic effects were greater. Concentration of contrast

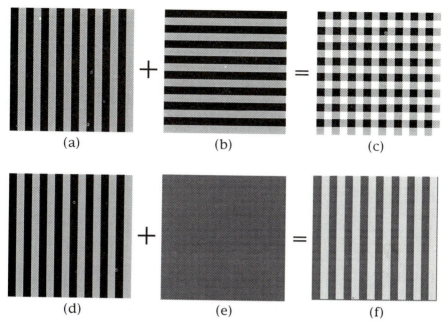

Fig. 2.8 (a, b, d) Vertical and horizontal gratings, and (c) the plaid pattern formed when the two are added optically. (f) The low-contrast grating that results when the vertical grating is replaced by a diffuse field (e) with the same space-averaged luminance.

energy in one dimension, as in gratings, appears to enhance the epileptogenic properties of a pattern.

Response to other pattern parameters

All susceptible patients show broadly similar effects of duty cycle and spatial frequency. The probability of epileptiform EEG activity is shown as a function of these variables in Figs 2.9 and 2.10. Patterns with a spatial frequency of 3 cycle deg^{-1} and a duty cycle of about 50 per cent are epileptogenic for most photosensitive patients. We will see later that the effects of spatial frequency depend on the angular radius of the pattern and its position in the visual field.

The differences between patients become apparent when the effects of other pattern characteristics are considered. Figure 2.11 shows the effects of pattern radius for patterns with a spatial frequency of 2 or 4 cycle deg^{-1}. It is immediately apparent that some photosensitive patients are sensitive to very small patterns whereas others become sensitive only when the pattern has a very large radius. The curves suggest thresholds that differ in terms of the total excitation required for epileptogenesis. We will return to this point later. For the present it is sufficient to note that for photosensitive patients as a group, the probability of epileptiform activity increases with a shallower slope than that for individual patients. The increase for the group is approximately linear when the pattern radius is plotted logarithmically, see Fig. 2.11, continuous line. This means that the increase is approximately linear with the total area of the pattern.

As might be anticipated, epileptiform EEG activity increases with the luminance of a pattern, as shown for one patient in Fig. 2.12(a). The data in this figure were obtained by Chatrian *et al.* (1970) using a technique in which a patient looked at a pattern of stripes continuously as the luminance was slowly increased. Figure 2.12(b) shows for a group of patients the probability of epileptiform EEG activity estimated from repeated randomized presentations. This technique provided data that were less stable than those in Fig. 2.12(a), although less activity was induced. Different patients have different thresholds below which no activity occurs, as was the case for the effects of pattern radius. Although most patients are sensitive in the photopic range of luminance where the cone receptors are active, some

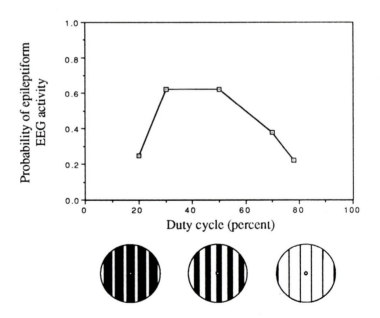

Fig. 2.9 The probability of epileptiform EEG activity as a function of the duty cycle of a pattern of stripes. The curve shows the mean for four patients. The patterns were black and white gratings, circular in outline, spatial frequency 3 cycle deg^{-1}, radius 12 deg, with a mean luminance of 3×10^2 cd m^{-2}, and a contrast of 7.5×10^{-1}. (After Wilkins *et al.* 1984.)

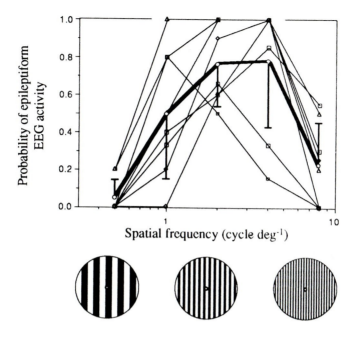

Fig. 2.10 The probability of epileptiform EEG activity as a function of the spatial frequency of a grating. The curves for eight patients are shown separately in grey and the bold curve shows the mean for the group, with the standard deviation of observations at each point shown by the bars. The patterns below the *x*-axis illustrate the change in spatial frequency schematically. The patterns were black and white gratings with square-wave luminance profile, circular in outline, radius 12 deg, with a mean luminance of 3×10^2 cd m^{-2}, and a contrast of 7.5×10^{-1}. (After Wilkins *et al.* 1979*a*.)

patients are still sensitive at very low luminance levels where only the rods are active. For the group as a whole, the increase is approximately linear with the logarithm of luminance. As can be seen from Fig. 2.12(b), the slope is such that a reduction in luminance by a factor of 10 is necessary to reduce the probability of epileptiform activity appreciably, except for a few patients sensitive only at high luminances.

Susceptibility increases with the luminance contrast between the stripes. Figure 2.13(a) shows data from Soso *et al.* (1980*b*) who measured the spike discharges occurring in 10 s presentations of square-wave gratings as contrast increased. The curves were obtained from one patient on different days and show the variation in sensitivity from day to day. Note that there appears to be little increase in epileptiform activity for pattern contrasts greater than 0.3.

Figure 2.13(b) shows data from Wilkins *et al.* (1979*a*, 1980) who observed the proportion of presentations on which discharges occurred, terminating observations upon the occurrence of such epileptiform activity. As with the effects of pattern size and pattern luminance, patients differ in the threshold contrast at which the activity first appears. The data for the group as a whole show an approximately linear increase with the logarithm of pattern contrast,

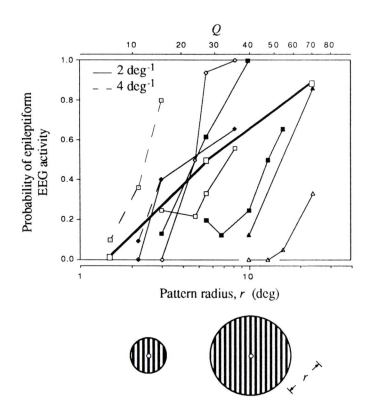

Fig. 2.11 The effects of the radius of a pattern of vertical stripes, circular in outline, with square-wave luminance profile (luminance contrast 7×10^{-1}, mean luminance 3×10^2 cd m^{-2}, and spatial frequency 2 or 4 cycle deg^{-1}, as indicated). Grey curves show data for seven patients, one of whom (solid squares) was tested twice. Note that the slope of the functions is broadly similar. Each has a different intercept, and for some patients the function appears to rise from a non-zero probability of epileptiform activity, perhaps signifying spontaneous activity. The bold curve shows the mean for the group and it has a shallower slope than that for individual patients. The diagrams below the x-axis show the increase in pattern size schematically and illustrate the pattern radius. The percentage area of visual cortex to which the pattern projects (Q) is also shown. (After Wilkins *et al.* 1979*a*.)

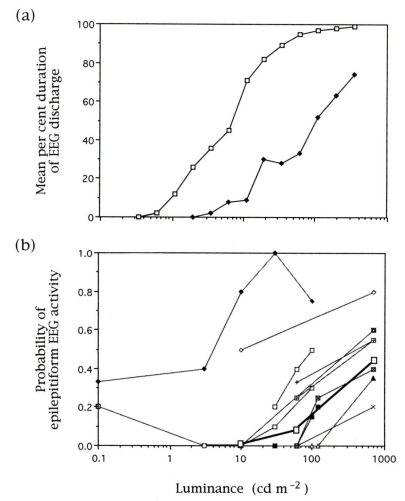

Fig. 2.12 The effects of the (space-averaged) luminance of a pattern of stripes. (a) Data from a single patient who looked at the pattern continuously with one eye (filled points) and both eyes (open points). (After Chatrian *et al.* 1970.) (b) Probability of epileptiform EEG activity. Curves for individual patients are shown by thin lines and the curve for the group is shown in bold. Each patient has a different threshold luminance below which no epileptiform activity occurs with the result that the average data for the group shows a shallower slope than that for individual patients. The stimuli were gratings with square-wave luminance profile and contrast 7×10^{-1}, circular in outline, radius varying so as to keep the probability less than 1.0 at high luminance. (After Wilkins *et al.* 1980.)

(a)

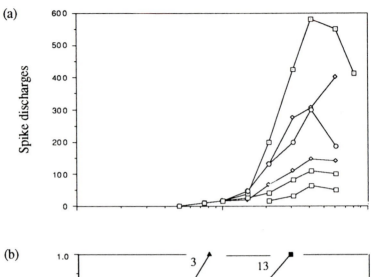

(b)

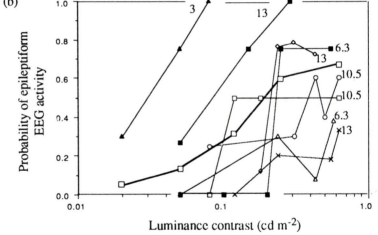

Luminance contrast (cd m^{-2})

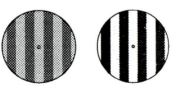

although this masks the non-linear increase that individuals may show. Again there is the suggestion of little increase in epileptiform activity for contrasts above 0.3.

If the stripes differ only in colour and not in photopic luminance they cease to be epileptogenic (Wilkins *et al.* 1980), except in a few patients with anomalous colour vision for whom the luminance is not matched (Wilkins, personal observations).

The orientation of the stripes usually has little effect. Figure 2.14 shows the average probability of epileptiform EEG activity for a group of eight patients, each of whom was examined with horizontal, vertical, and oblique stripes. The figure also shows the data from one individual for whom there was a significant effect of orientation that could not be attributed to focusing aberrations (astigmatism). Similar data from a patient examined by Soso *et al.* (1980c) are also shown.

Susceptibility is reduced when the pattern is moved continuously across the stripes in one direction. If the direction of movement is rapidly and repeatedly changed, however, susceptibility is *enhanced* rather than reduced. The enhancement is considerable. Many patients are sensitive to oscillating patterns and about 20 per cent of patients are not at all sensitive to stationary patterns. Figure 2.15 shows data obtained from such patients (Binnie *et al.* 1979a). It can be seen the spatial and temporal characteristics have independent effects. The worst frequency of oscillation is 20 Hz regardless of spatial frequency, and the worst spatial frequency is about 2 cycle deg^{-1}, regardless of oscillation frequency.

2.2.3 Viewing conditions

Epileptic visual sensitivity is usually greatest under conditions of binocular stimulation. Covering one eye eliminated the photoconvulsive response to flicker in 164 of the 244 patients seen by Jeavons and Harding (1975, p. 73). In most of the remainder the response was attenuated and only 2 per

---

Fig. 2.13 The effects of the luminance contrast of a striped pattern. The contrast is defined according to Fig. 2.6. (a) The number of spike discharges recorded from one patient whilst the pattern was fixated. The curves were obtained on different days and reflect the variation in sensitivity from day to day. (After Soso *et al.* 1980b.) (b) Probability of epileptiform EEG activity. Data from seven patients, one of whom (solid squares) was tested twice; mean of all patients shown in bold. The patterns had a spatial frequency of 2 cycle deg^{-1}, a mean luminance of 3×10^2 cd m^{-2}, and were circular in outline. The radius (shown beside each curve) was adjusted according to the sensitivity of the patient at the outset of testing in an attempt to keep the probability low when the contrast was high. The diagrams below the *x*-axis show the increase in contrast schematically. (After Wilkins *et al.* 1980.)

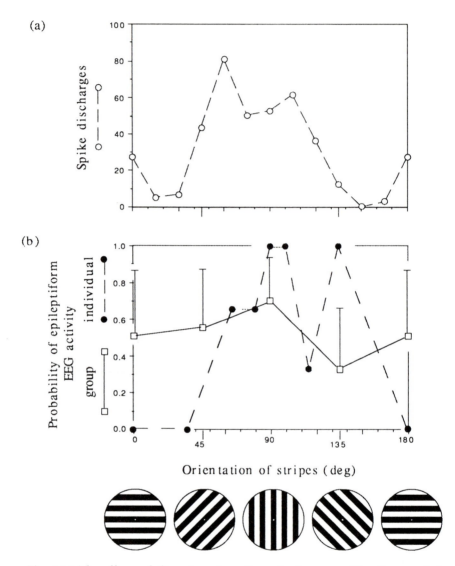

Fig. 2.14 The effects of the orientation of a striped pattern. The diagrams below the *x*-axis show the orientation schematically. (a) The number of spike discharges in a single patient in response to a pattern with various orientations. (After Soso *et al.* 1980*c*.) (b) The probability of epileptiform EEG activity as a function of pattern orientation. The solid curve shows the mean for a group of eight patients, with the standard deviation of observations at each point. The broken grey curve shows the data for one individual who was not astigmatic. The patterns had square-wave luminance profile, mean luminance 3×10^2 cd m^{-2}, contrast 7×10^{-1}, and were circular in outline, with radius 12 deg. (After Wilkins *et al.* 1979*a*.)

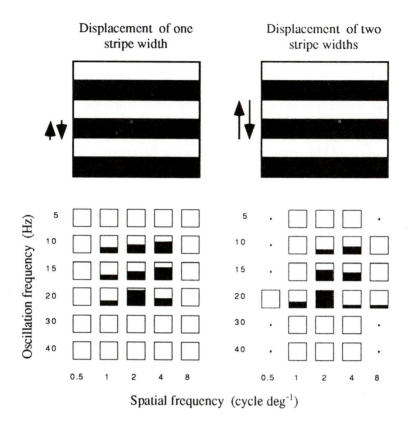

Fig. 2.15 The effects of spatial and temporal frequency for oscillating patterns. The probability of epileptiform EEG activity is shown by the proportion of each rectangle filled. The patterns were rear projected via a mirror moving with a triangular profile of angular position vs time, i.e. at constant velocity with abrupt reversals of direction. They had a contrast of at least 80 per cent, a 50 per cent duty cycle, and subtended about 5 deg. (After Binnie *et al.* 1979*a*.)

cent showed a similar response with binocular and monocular stimulation. Pattern sensitivity is also reduced by covering one eye (Chatrian *et al.* 1970; Wilkins *et al.* 1979*a*, 1980).

2.2.4 Common environmental stimuli

One of the most potent precipitants of seizures is probably sunlight interrupted by road-side trees. Discotheque stroboscopes are another source of danger. One of the most widely available sources of epileptogenic stimulation, however, is the television, particularly a set with a large screen viewed from less than 1 m. A large proportion of patients with photosensitive epilepsy suffer their first seizure when watching television, and many suffer seizures only under these circumstances. When television-induced seizures were first described they were attributed to the malfunction of the set which was common in the early days of television, when the picture would frequently become unstable and 'roll', introducing a low-frequency flicker (Livingston 1952). As the number of reports increased it became apparent that seizures could be induced by a set that was functioning quite normally. The details why are given in the section on television epilepsy in Chapter 7, together with techniques for avoiding television-induced seizures.

Seizures induced by computer display terminals are rare, but they do occur. The characteristics of computer displays differ a great deal, and most are unlikely to provoke a seizure. Unfortunately some displays, particularly those used in British schools, closely resemble conventional television and are just as likely to provoke seizures. The differences between displays and their relevance for epilepsy and headaches are discussed in Chapter 7.

2.2.5 Measuring susceptibility – theoretical implications

The stimulus characteristics of patterns that induce the epileptiform EEG response are of interest for both practical and theoretical reasons. By studying the patterns that are likely to induce the response it is possible to learn which patterns in the environment are likely to be a danger to the patient. The characteristics of such patterns are also of theoretical significance. Recent advances in our understanding of the neurophysiological processes involved in pattern vision can be combined with a knowledge of the stimulus characteristics responsible for pattern sensitive epilepsy and provide clues regarding the nature of the epileptic process, as will be shown in the next section.

2.3 Inferences regarding the seizure mechanism

The characteristics of patterns that elicit epileptiform EEG activity enable inferences to be drawn concerning the seizure mechanism. These inferences will now be reviewed. The evidence for each will be considered in turn, together with the way in which the inference is drawn. For the benefit of those readers who do not wish to consider the evidence in detail, a very straightforward summary is possible:

In patients with photosensitive epilepsy, the seizures start in the visual cortex of one cerebral hemisphere, or in both hemispheres independently. The hemispheres can have very different convulsive thresholds, even in patients with epilepsy of the idiopathic generalized type. The seizures occur when normal physiological excitation involves more than a critical cortical area, but is likely only when the excitation is rhythmic. The antiepileptic drug, sodium valproate, prevents the spread of the discharge, but does not affect the mechanisms that trigger it.

We now consider each of the statements in the above summary and the evidence upon which it is based.

2.3.1 Pattern-induced epilepsy starts in the visual cortex

There are several lines of evidence for a cortical trigger mechanism. The first three relate to the stimulus characteristics of patterns responsible for the discharge, and the last two the characteristics of the response they evoke.

Stimulus characteristics

As we saw in Section 2.2, the longer the length of line contour within the pattern the more likely a discharge is to occur (the pattern in Fig. 2.16(a) is less epileptogenic than that in Fig. 2.16(b), and the pattern in Fig. 2.16(b) less epileptogenic than that in Figure 2.16(c); see Wilkins *et al.* 1979*a*, 1980). The effect of the length of line contour suggests a role is played by neurones in the visual cortex. As was demonstrated first by Hubel and Wiesel, these neurones respond to linear contours: lines and edges (Hubel 1988).

If the two eyes see different patterns (e.g. the left eye sees the pattern shown in Fig. 2.16(d) and the right eye the pattern in Fig. 2.16(e) the discharge is less likely than when both eyes see the same pattern and binocular fusion occurs (Wilkins *et al.* 1979*a*). Many neurones in the visual cortex respond to stimulation of either eye, and some respond more vigorously to binocular than to monocular stimulation. The fact that epileptiform EEG activity occurs mainly under binocular stimulation is therefore consistent with the idea that seizures are triggered in the visual cortex. If only one eye sees the pattern, the response is less than when both eyes do, presumably because the cortical excitation is reduced.

As mentioned in Section 2.2, a few patients are sensitive only when a pattern of stripes is oriented at particular angles, for example they may be sensitive to the pattern in Fig. 2.16(e) but not to the patterns in Figs 2.16(d) or (f) (Chatrian *et al.* 1970; Wilkins *et al.* 1979*a*). This orientation selectivity is not due simply to poor focusing at one orientation: the eyes may show no evidence of *astigmatism* and yet the patient may be sensitive only to a limited range of pattern orientations. Neurones in the visual cortex respond selectively to line contours with a limited range of orientations, and so the fact that patients can show a selective response to certain pattern orientations is consistent with a trigger mechanism involving neurones in the visual cortex.

Response characteristics

The EEG response to intermittent light is often generalized, but when this generalized response is suppressed with sodium valproate then focal activity remains at the back of the head, over the visual cortex (Darby *et al*. 1986).

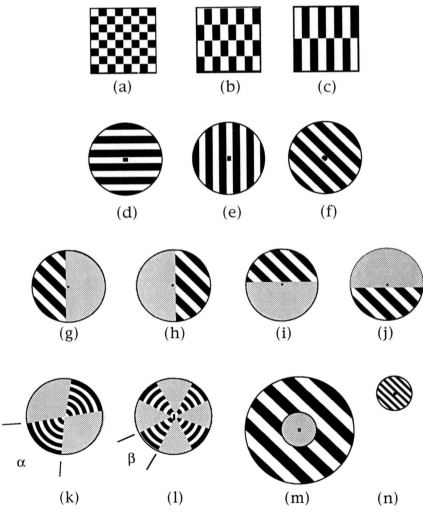

Fig. 2.16 Patterns used in an investigation of pattern-sensitive epilepsy. The diagrams are not to scale. For patterns (k) and (l) the sector angles α and β were adjusted to suit the sensitivity of the patient.

The EEG response to pattern can be even more localized. The distribution of the electrical activity on the surface of the scalp depends on the localization of the pattern with respect to the centre of gaze. The neuronal wiring between the eye and the brain is such that the visual world to the right of the centre of gaze is analysed by the left cerebral hemisphere, and the right hemisphere analyses the left visual field. The response to patterns that occupy the left visual field (e.g. Fig. 2.16(g) is maximal over the right posterior part of the head, and the opposite is true for patterns in the right visual field (e.g. Fig. 2.16(h); Soso *et al.* 1980c; Wilkins *et al.* 1981). In some patients the response to patterns that occupy the upper and lower visual fields (e.g. Figs 2.16(i) and (j)) shows a dissociation along the vertical midline (Wilkins *et al.* 1981). That is, patterns in the upper field show a lower response than those in the lower field, and vice versa. In short, the positioning of epileptiform EEG activity over the surface of the scalp follows the underlying visual cortex.

The electrical activity measured at the scalp depends on the position of the electrodes with respect to the electrical field from the neuronal activity. Although, as we have seen, neurones buried in the calcarine fissure may produce electrical activity on the opposite (contralateral) side of the head, more anterior visual areas lie near the surface of the brain and are unlikely to produce such anomalous lateralization. The appearance of epileptiform EEG activity over the cerebral hemisphere that is presumably active suggests that the neuronal discharge responsible is not confined within the calcarine fissure: anterior visual areas are presumably involved.

2.3.2 The epilepsy involves one cerebral hemisphere or both hemispheres independently

In some patients, pattern-evoked epileptiform activity may be more pronounced when the pattern is presented in the left visual field, in other patients the opposite is the case (Wilkins *et al.* 1981). For example, the pattern in Fig. 2.16(g) may be more epileptogenic than that in Fig. 2.16(h), or vice versa. The different sensitivity to left-sided and right-sided patterns seems to arise from different excitability of the visual cortex of the two halves of the brain. For example, when the left visual stimulus is more likely to evoke a response, it is because the right cerebral hemisphere is more hyperexcitable. Such an explanation is supported by another observation: when the pattern sensitivity is greater to patterns on one side of the centre of gaze, the patient's EEG response to bilateral stimulation (e.g. from diffuse intermittent light) shows a slight asymmetry. For example, if the sensitivity is greatest for patterns in the right visual field, then the EEG response has a slightly higher amplitude over the left side of the head and may involve more electrodes on this side (Binnie *et al.* 1981). This evidence for an unbalanced hyperexcitability of the two cerebral hemispheres is common not only in patients with partial or symptomatic generalized epilepsy, but also those with epilepsy of the idiopathic generalized type.

Many patients do not show any cerebral asymmetry. Nevertheless, even in these patients it is possible to infer that the hemispheres act independently in triggering the epileptiform activity. This inference is based on three lines of evidence.

First, as has already been shown, the response to a pattern presented in one visual half-field occurs on the opposite side, over the area of the brain that the pattern stimulates, perhaps confined within the contralateral hemisphere.

Second, when the pattern is presented in one lateral visual half-field the response is far more likely than when the same size pattern is presented in the upper or lower visual half-field (see Figs 2.16(i) and (j)), and is therefore presented to both hemispheres. Perhaps a critical amount of excitation within one hemisphere is necessary to induce the discharge.

Third, if a pattern is presented in both visual fields (e.g. Fig. 2.16(f)), the probability of a discharge is not much greater than when the pattern is presented in only one half-field (e.g. Figs 2.16(g) and (h)). In other words, a much larger bilateral pattern stimulating both hemispheres is not much more epileptogenic than a unilateral pattern, half the area, that stimulates only one. Under other circumstances, doubling the area of a pattern increases the probability of epileptiform EEG activity appreciably, see Fig. 2.11. The cerebral hemispheres appear to act independently in the induction of the epileptiform activity. Such a finding would be expected if a critical amount of excitation within a hemisphere were necessary for the discharge.

The above evidence is quite consistent with the view that the seizures arise in the visual cortex. There are very few interactions between the hemispheres in the posterior visual areas of the brain: those that there are simply serve to 'sew together' the two halves of the visual field. It is mainly in more anterior visual areas in the temporal lobe that appreciable interhemispheric interactions occur, and cells can be excited by stimulation in either lateral visual half-field (Zeki 1970, 1978, 1980). The evidence for an independent activation of epileptic activity within each hemisphere suggests that the activity is triggered only or mainly by neural mechanisms in more posterior visual areas, but not, as we have seen, those confined within the calcarine fissure.

2.3.3 The seizures are started by normal physiological excitation

The inference that seizures are triggered by normal excitation is based on the fact that photosensitive patients have normal vision (normal acuity, normal stereopsis, heterophoria, etc.). It is rare to find ophthalmological abnormalities except in patients with symptomatic generalized epilepsy. What is more surprising is that contrast sensitivity is normal. Contrast sensitivity refers to the ability to see very faint patterns of stripes. Soso *et al.* (1980*b*) reported normal contrast sensitivity in two pattern-sensitive patients using a 'yellow – green' oscilloscope display. We have also examined contrast sensitivity (under white light) and found it to be normal. We used the Cambridge Low Contrast Gratings, a test developed for this purpose. (The test can detect subtle visual deficits in circumstances where conventional ophthalmological tests fail to do so. It has revealed impairments in a variety of diseases, including optic neuritis, multiple sclerosis, diabetes, and glaucoma (Wilkins *et al.* 1988). The test consists of a booklet viewed from 6 m. The patient is required to choose which of two pages in the booklet contains the grating, and the gratings get fainter and fainter.) Photosensitive patients tend to score well within the norms for their age. In general, therefore, patients have perfectly normal vision for patterns that would elicit epileptiform activity were they of higher contrast.

2.3.4 The seizures start when physiological excitation involves more than a critical cortical area

Any region of visual cortex will induce epileptiform abnormalities provided a sufficient area is stimulated. We can infer this for two related reasons.

1. Very different patterns of sectored concentric rings have a similar capacity to elicit epileptiform EEG abnormalities, provided the total areas of the patterns are similar. For example, patterns with two large sectors, such as Fig. 2.16(k), have the same effect as patterns with four sectors of half the angular size, such as Fig. 2.16(l). When the probability of an EEG response is plotted as a function of pattern area, curves for the various types of pattern simply overlap, see Fig. 2.17.

2. The sectored rings shown in Figs 2.16(k) and (l) are laterally symmetric and stimulate both hemispheres equivalently. They also distribute the excitation equivalently on the central and peripheral visual field. If, however, the pattern is such as to stimulate only the periphery, the probability of epileptiform activity is reduced: a large patterned annulus (Fig. 2.16(m)) has the same effect as a small disc that stimulates central vision (Fig. 2.16(n)). This would appear to be because more of the visual cortex is devoted to analysis of central vision than the periphery. A simple formula due to Drasdo (1977) expresses the percentage of cortex devoted to analysis of a circular region of the visual field. When gaze is directed at the centre of the region and the radius is increased, the percentage of the cortex to which the region projects increases as Q, shown in Fig. 2.11. Figure 2.11 also shows the radius of the pattern, r, for comparison.

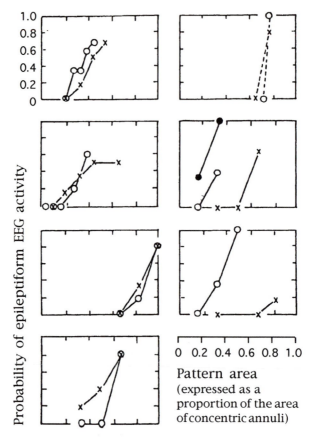

Fig. 2.17 Probability of epileptiform activity in response to stripes formed from concentric annuli cut in sectors and opposed diametrically (as in Fig 2.16(k) and (l)). Each graph shows data from an individual patient. The circles are for patterns with two sectors and the crosses for patterns with four. (After Wilkins *et al.* 1980.)

A group of patients was examined using various patterned annuli and patterned discs and the area of the patterns was increased until epileptiform EEG activity just appeared (Wilkins *et al.* 1980). Each point in Fig. 2.18(a) represents a patient and the position is determined by the area of the disc and the area of the annulus at which the EEG activity occurred. The points are widely dispersed. In general, patients were less susceptible to the annuli, but to an extent that varied with the particular dimensions. When the points were replotted according to the percentage area of visual cortex to which the patterns projected, Q, the points lay scattered either side of the diagonal, see Fig. 2.18(b). This indicates that the annuli and the discs had similar effects provided they stimulated a similar area of the visual cortex.

The ability to see fine detail is poorer in the periphery, and, as might be expected, the effects of spatial frequency differ for annuli and discs. As can be seen from Fig. 2.18(c), the spatial frequency at which annuli are most likely to induce epileptiform EEG activity is lower than that for discs. No allowance for this difference was made in Fig. 2.18(b), and if it had been, the scatter might have been further reduced. The x-axis in Fig. 2.11 gives the area of discs of stripes together with values of Q. The probability of epileptiform activity for the group of patients as a whole increases linearly with Q.

The increase in epileptiform activity with the area of visual cortex stimulated suggests that the activity is a response to the number of neurones excited by the pattern. Such a viewpoint would be consistent with the effects of pattern contrast shown in Fig. 2.13. because at contrasts above 0.3 most cortical neurones have saturated or begun to do so (Movshon *et al.* 1978). Note that there is little increase in epileptiform activity for pattern contrasts above 0.3.

2.3.5 The seizures are most likely when cortical excitation is rhythmic

The movement of a pattern has very pronounced effects on its epileptic properties. These effects lead to important inferences regarding the role of the temporal characteristics of excitation in the generation of the epileptic response (Binnie *et al.* 1985).

Drifting patterns

Patterns that drift continuously in one direction are extremely unlikely to evoke epileptiform activity. Usually, when the eyes look at drifting patterns they have a tendency to follow the motion of the pattern, and then jerk back, producing *optokinetic nystagmus*. Any such nystagmus would interfere with comparisons of different types of pattern motion. Fortunately the nystagmus can be avoided if gaze is directed at a central point and a bilateral pattern of stripes drifts continuously towards that point from either side (leftwards in the right visual field and rightwards in the left, see Fig. 2.19(a)). Stable gaze can then be achieved. Under these circumstances, epileptiform EEG activity is very unlikely to occur at any drift velocity.

Vibrating and phase-reversing patterns

Although epileptiform EEG activity is so unlikely in response to a drifting pattern, a small change in the characteristics of the motion can make the pattern very likely to provoke such activity. The change involves the direction of pattern movement: not its velocity. If the pattern repeatedly

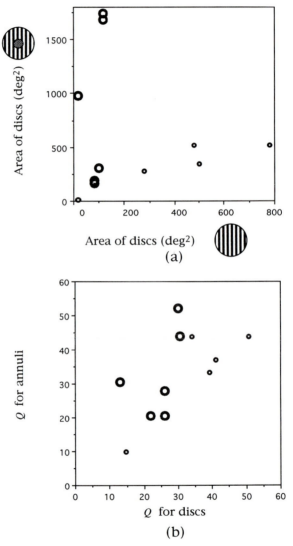

Fig. 2.18 (a) Epileptiform EEG activity in response to patterns of stripes that are complete discs or that have a central circular section removed to form an annulus. The outer radius of the pattern was increased until epileptiform activity just appeared; the inner radius was large or small, as indicated by the size of the point. Each point represents a patient and its position is determined by the area of the disc and annulus for which epileptiform activity first appeared. (b) The same data as in (a) replotted using instead of pattern area, the percentage area of cortex to which the pattern projected, Q.

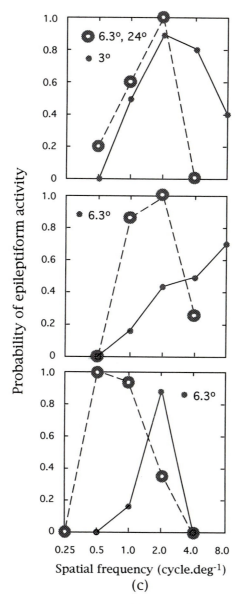

Fig. 2.18 (*cont.*) (c) Curves showing the probability of epileptiform EEG activity as a function of spatial frequency for discs (radius 3 degrees or 6.3 degrees, as shown) and for annuli (inner radius 6.3 degrees, outer radius 24 degrees). (After Wilkins *et al.* 1980.)

drifts at a constant velocity through a distance of one or two stripe widths before abruptly reversing its direction of movement, epileptiform EEG activity is readily provoked. The pattern is most epileptogenic when 10–20 reversals are made every second, see Fig. 2.15.

The pattern is also highly epileptogenic if it remains stationary but reverses in contrast (white stripes changing to black: black to white) 10–20 times per second.

Static patterns

Static patterns are more epileptogenic than drifting patterns. The only retinal movement from a static pattern is that which results from the small drifts and flicks that the eyes make during fixation.

These effects of pattern movement can easily be explained and they provide important insights into epilepsy.

Pattern contours pass through the overlapping receptive fields of cortical neurones causing them to fire. Whilst the pattern is moving in one direction, contours flow into and out of overlapping receptive fields causing those neurones that are sensitive to that particular direction of motion to fire, see Fig. 2.19(c). Therefore the population of neurones as a whole presumably shows a sustained excitation. Some neurones are directionally sensitive, and fire mainly in response to only one direction of motion. Every time the pattern changes direction some of the neurones should increase firing, others should decrease. If the pattern changes direction rhythmically, as it does when it is oscillated, then the population of neurones as a whole will show rhythmic excitation, see Fig. 2.19(d). Similar rhythmic excitation should occur in response to a phase-reversing pattern. No rhythmic response of the neuronal population should result from a drifting pattern – just a continuous excitation. Stationary patterns are more potent than drifting patterns presumably because the small movements that the eyes make when they are gazing at a point are sufficient to synchronize the action of some neurones.

Synchronization of neural activity has long been known to be characteristic of the epileptic discharge. It is responsible for the EEG waveforms of the photoconvulsive response. The effects of pattern movement suggest that synchronization is necessary at the very outset of the epileptic discharge, and is not simply a reflection of the later activity.

2.3.6 Sodium valproate prevents the spread of the discharge

The characteristics of pattern sensitivity also give some insights into the action of the drugs that are used to control epilepsy. One of the most effective drugs for controlling visually induced seizures is sodium valproate, and as we shall see in Chapter 3, this drug has now been shown to be

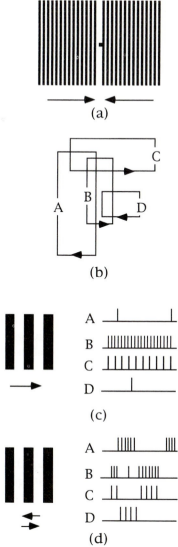

Fig. 2.19 Schematic diagram of various categories of pattern motion, and the neural consequences of that motion. (a) A bipartite pattern, each half drifting towards a central fixation point. (b) The overlapping rectangles represent the receptive fields of visual neurones labelled A–D, and the arrowheads the direction of motion to which they preferentially respond. Beneath are two schematic diagrams of moving patterns, the arrows giving the direction of motion. Beside each diagram are illustrations of the way in which the neurones A–D might respond to that motion. The continuous motion of a pattern in one direction (c) might be expected to give rise to continuous activity in those neurones that respond to the direction of movement, and perhaps to a reduction in the spontaneous activity of other neurones. Vibratory motion across the contours of the pattern (d) should give rise to a rhythmic and partially synchronized pattern of activity in the nerve network taken as a whole.

successful in the prevention of migraine. It is thought to affect the availability of the inhibitory *neurotransmitter* γ-aminobutyric acid (GABA), although the mechanisms of its action remain obscure (Meldrum and Wilkins 1984). (A neurotransmitter is a chemical that carries a message across the junctions between neurones.)

It is desirable to adjust the dose of a drug to the minimum necessary for seizure control. This is often done over the course of several months, gradually increasing the dose from time to time if seizures continue, and gradually reducing the dose if the patient has been free of seizures for a long time. A group of pattern-sensitive patients was examined over a period of two years whilst the dose of valproate was adjusted in this way. Pattern sensitivity was assessed during an EEG recorded immediately before each change of dose (Darby *et al.* 1986).

As the dose of sodium valproate increased there was a decrease in the duration of the EEG discharge, its voltage, the number of electrodes it involved, and the number of component waveforms (spikes, sharp waves, slow waves).

During the EEG examination patients were shown patterns of stripes that gradually increased in size until the discharge occurred. Although the discharge decreased in the manner described above, the critical pattern size just sufficient to induce the discharge showed relatively little change. The probability of a discharge was reduced, but when the discharge occurred it did so in response to the same pattern size. This would suggest that, although sodium valproate affected the spread of the discharge, the physiological mechanisms responsible for triggering the discharge were not so markedly affected.

In the chapters that follow, it will be shown that epileptogenic patterns are uncomfortable to look at, not necessarily for patients with epilepsy, but for those who suffer eye-strain and headaches. it may therefore be significant that valproate has been shown to prevent migraine in a double-blind study (Hering and Kuritzky 1992).

2.3.7 Underlying pathophysiology

This chapter has reviewed some of the physiological mechanisms responsible for the visual induction of seizures. The seizures are triggered when normal physiological excitation in the visual cortex of one hemisphere is rhythmic (synchronized) and exceeds some 'critical mass'.

Recordings from single units and staining techniques have revealed that the visual cortex is organized into columns of cells responsive to bars and edges with particular orientation. The orientation selectively is due to inhibition from a network of interneurones that use an inhibitory neurotransmitter GABA (Sillito 1979). A visual stimulus such as a grating is likely to result in patches of localized excitation of (pyramidal) neurones, those that respond to the particular grating orientation. A strong localized excitation may deplete the local availability of inhibitory neurotransmitter, particularly if the excitation is synchronized. This may have no consequences normally, but if there is a minimal and diffuse failure of inhibition in patients with photosensitive epilepsy (as hypothesized by Meldrum and Wilkins 1984), the depletion of inhibitory neurotransmitter may lead to hyperexcitability, and the spread of a neural discharge in response to strong stimulation. The visual stimulation can therefore be seen as further stressing an already compromised system of cortical inhibition.

In this chapter we have concentrated on the visual precipitation of seizures. We have seen that seizures result when cortical stimulation is 'massive', localized, and synchronized. In the chapters that follow we will see that such physiological excitation can have adverse consequences not just for those with epilepsy, but for many others as well.

3   Illusions and headaches

Certain geometric patterns can be uncomfortable to look at and may some-times provoke anomalous visual effects: illusions of colour, shape, and motion. The stimuli responsible are very similar to those that provoke seizures in patients with photosensitive epilepsy. Susceptibility to discomfort and anomalous visual effects varies considerably from one observer to another and is greatest in those who suffer frequent severe headaches, especially prior to headache onset, or after exposure to a virus. Susceptibility to patterns is particularly pronounced in people suffering from migraine. In migraine with aura, the illusions predominate in the affected visual field.

The previous chapter concerned the way in which visual stimulation elicits seizures, the nature of the stimulation, and some of the physiological mechanisms whereby the seizures are induced. In the present chapter it is shown that similar visual stimulation can induce a variety of other effects in people without epilepsy. These effects can be both visuo-perceptual (anomalous perceptual effects of various kinds), or they can be somatic: eye-ache, headache, nausea. The visuo-perceptual effects are related to the somatic effects in a variety of ways.

3.1 Anomalous visuo-perceptual effects

The pattern of stripes shown in the frontispiece can provoke a variety of anomalous visuo-perceptual effects: illusions of colour, shape, and motion. Do not look at the pattern if you have photosensitive epilepsy or migraine. After observing the dot in the centre of the pattern for a few seconds most people report that the lines appear to shimmer. Some people also see colours, and a shadowy rhomboid lattice. Others may observe the pattern for a long time without seeing anything anomalous. In short, some people are far more susceptible to anomalous perceptual effects than others. There are also large differences in susceptibility to the non-visual effects. Most people find the pattern rather unpleasant to look at, but a few find it quite unbearable and see many distortions. As we will see, the people who find the pattern aversive usually report distortions and they are usually those who suffer migraine.

 Provided you do not yourself have epilepsy or migraine, you can judge your own susceptibility by looking at the pattern in the frontispiece. Look at the dot at the centre of the pattern for 5 s (counting to yourself). Then look away and tick off the illusions you saw on the check list opposite. If you find the pattern highly aversive, do not force yourself to look at it. If you have photosensitive epilepsy or migraine, do not look at the pattern.

Check list:

> red
> green
> blue
> yellow
> blurring
> bending of the lines
> shadowy shapes amongst the lines
> shimmering of the lines
> flickering of the whole pattern
>
> nausea
> dizziness
> pain

Try and describe the various effects you see simply in terms of the above list. Do not look at the pattern for more than a few seconds. If you have to tick more than two illusions in the above list you are more sensitive than average and you should avoid looking at the pattern for a long time.

3.2 Origin of the anomalous perceptual effects

The origin of the perceptual effects seen in patterns of stripes such as the pattern in the frontispiece is still unclear despite a long history of investigation. Most of the perceptual effects were first described in the last century. 'During intense viewing of the parallel lines of an engraving one observes an oscillation of the lines which on closer inspection involves some being closer together and others farther apart, so that the lines appear in the form of waves' Purkinje (1823, p. 122). 'If the eye looks at (parallel black lines drawn upon white paper) steadily and continuously, the black lines soon lose their straightness and parallelism, and inclose luminous spaces somewhat like the links of a number of parallel chains. When this change takes place, the eye which sees it experiences a good deal of uneasiness, an effect which is communicated to the eye which is shut. When this dazzling effect takes place the luminous spaces between the lines become coloured, some with yellow and others with green and blue light' (Brewster 1832, p. 170). Wade (1977) has reviewed the descriptions of the anomalous perceptual effects seen in patterns of stripes and some of the possible ocular mechanisms. A wide variety of mechanisms has been proposed involving:

(1) the small movements that eyes make during fixation;

(2) changes in the focusing power of the lens of the eye;

(3) the fact that light at the 'red end' of the visible spectrum is bent by the lens less than light at the 'blue end' and is therefore focused in a different plane.

Although these peripheral mechanisms may explain some of the illusions, there remain certain effects that defy explanation in these terms. Take, for example, the shadowy lattice of rhomboid shapes that is sometimes seen

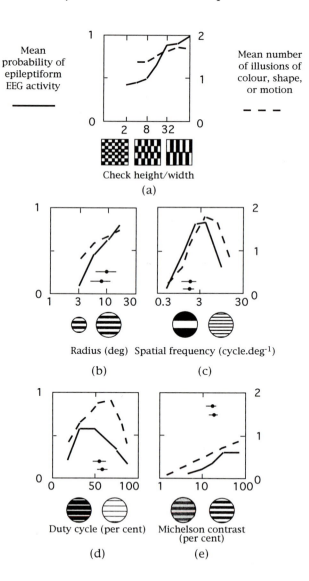

in pastel shades of colour forming a background to a striped pattern, or the tiny dots seen streaming in a direction orthogonal to the lines. These illusions have a structure that can be attributed more readily to inhibitory connections in the visual cortex, as suggested by Georgeson (1976, 1980).

The illusions of one type tend to occur with those of another. Observers who see colour usually report illusions of shape and motion as well. As already mentioned, the colours tend to have a spatial structure of their own, often resembling a rhomboid lattice. The patterns that induce one type of illusion are also those that induce the other types. For example, the patterns that induce illusions of motion are also those that induce illusions of colour and shape. As will shortly become clear, it is parsimonious to take account of these co-occurrences and attribute the various perceptual anomalies to a common cortical mechanism.

3.3 Links between illusions and seizures

3.3.1 Patterns·

In a series of experiments, groups of normal observers were asked to look at a pattern for a period of a few seconds (usually 10 s) and to report the illusions they saw (Wilkins *et al.* 1984). The observers described the

---

Fig. 3.1(left) The mean number of illusions seen in a pattern of stripes, and the probability with which the pattern will induce epileptiform EEG abnormalities in patients with photosensitive epilepsy, expressed as functions of the spatial parameters of the pattern. (a) Effects of line length/width ratio. (b) Effects of pattern size (angular subtense of the radius of the pattern at the eye). (c) Effects of spatial frequency (number of spatial cycles of the pattern in one degree subtended at the eye). (d) Effects of duty cycle (proportion of spatial cycle occupied by bright bars). (e) Effects of Michelson contrast (difference in the luminance of the bright and dark sections of the pattern expressed as a proportion of their sum). The icons beneath the x-axis show how variations in the parameter affect the appearance of the pattern. Some of the data were collected with patterns that had a different orientation. Pattern orientation had no general effect, although some patients exhibited greater sensitivity to certain orientations. The curves were obtained by manipulating each parameter independently. The values of the other parameters were chosen arbitrarily, but as the data were acquired it transpired that the values chosen were close to those for which illusions and epileptiform EEG activity were maximally likely. The pair of horizontal lines with central point in each figure show respectively the range of values and the mean for printed text, where the text is considered as a pattern of striped lines, see Chapter 5. The upper of the two lines refers to text rated as 'clear', and the lower to 'less clear' text. (After Wilkins *et al.* 1984; Wilkins and Nimmo-Smith 1987)

illusions by checking items on a list similar to the one in the previous section. Figure 3.1 shows the mean number of illusions reported as a function of various pattern parameters. The x-axis of each graph shows the pattern parameter that was varied and beneath the axis are icons demonstrating the effects of the variation. Only one pattern parameter was varied at a time; the other pattern characteristics remained constant. The values of these constant parameters were chosen arbitrarily, but as data were collected it transpired that in every case the choice was close to that for which illusions were maximally likely.

The solid lines in Fig. 3.1 show the probability of epileptiform EEG activity in patients with pattern-sensitive epilepsy. The probability was estimated by showing patterns in random order for several trials and noting the occurrence of any epileptiform EEG activity, as described in Section 2.2. It can be seen from Fig. 3.1 that the illusions are induced by patterns very similar to those that evoke epileptiform EEG activity. Both illusions and epileptiform activity are most likely:

(1) when the pattern is striped (that is, when it is unidimensional and has a square-wave luminance profile): the longer the stripes the greater the illusions, and the greater the chances of epileptiform EEG activity;

(2) when the entire pattern is large (when it subtends an angle of at least 3 degrees at the eye);

(3) when each stripe subtends about 15 min of arc at the eye (i.e. when the spatial frequency is about 3 cycle $\deg^{-1}$);

(4) when the stripes have even width and spacing (a duty cycle of 50 per cent);

(5) when the stripes are alternately bright and dark (when the pattern has a high contrast);

(6) when the pattern is viewed with both eyes rather than monocularly.

In all the above respects, the pattern characteristics likely to produce anomalous visual effects are also those likely to produce epileptiform EEG activity in patients with photosensitive epilepsy.

The parallels between illusions and epilepsy do not end here. Figures 2.16(k) – (n) show a variety of other striped patterns in which size has been varied in a number of ways. In Figs 2.16(k) and (l) the stripes are formed from concentric rings cut as per the slices of a cake with the sectors diametrically opposed. The pattern size can be increased by increasing the number of sectors or their angular size. In the patterned annulus shown in Fig. 2.16(m), size can be increased by decreasing the internal diameter or increasing the external. It will be recalled from Section 2.3.4 that the probability of epileptiform EEG activity is proportional to the area of visual cortex to which the pattern projects. Figure 3.2 shows the mean number of illusions as a function of this area separately for each pattern type. It will be seen that the number of reported illusions increases with cortical projection, although patterns of linear stripes produce slightly more illusions than those with curvilinear contours, presumably because cortical 'line detectors' are involved.

In summary, changing the size of a pattern by varying the number or angular size of diametrically opposed sectors, or by varying the size of central or peripheral sections has an effect on illusions that mirrors the effect on epileptiform EEG activity. For such patterns the likelihood of both illusions and epileptiform activity is determined simply by the area of the cortex to which the pattern projects (see Section 2.3.4).

Although the illusions and epileptiform activity are determined by the cortical projection, this is true for symmetrical patterns only. Note that the patterns shown in Fig. 3.2 are symmetrical either side of the centre. Some people see more illusions to the left or right of the centre of gaze, i.e. the illusions predominate in the left or right visual field. Similarly, some patients with pattern-sensitive epilepsy are more likely to show epileptiform EEG activity in one lateral visual field than in the other (see Section 2.3.2). These findings suggest that the cerebral hemispheres differ in susceptibility. The hemispheric differences are not reflected in the measurements made using the symmetrical patterns in Fig. 3.2.

3.3.2 Flicker

Illusions of colour have long been known to occur in response to diffuse flicker (Bidwell 1896) and to moving patterns of stripes, particularly those on the Benham top, a disc bearing a sectored pattern and exhibiting colours when rotated (Benham 1894). The colours are usually attributed to different time-constants of the photoreceptors (Cohen and Gordon 1949), but it is unclear how this explanation accounts for the considerable individual differences in what is seen under given conditions. The illusions of colour occur at frequencies that are the most epileptogenic, compare Fig. 2.3 with Fig. 3.3.

There are also illusions of form that appear when a diffuse field is flickered. In two observers, Young *et al.* (1975) described grids and honeycomb illusions, the former most readily induced at about 10 Hz and the latter at about 20 Hz, the strength depending to some extent on the observer.

The links between illusions and epilepsy are not confined to pattern characteristics, but extend to the physiological state of the observer. Both illusions and the likelihood of seizures increase after sleep deprivation (Wilkins *et al.* 1984).

Although the similarities between the patterns that provoke illusions and those that provoke epileptiform EEG activity are impressive, there are two instructive differences. It will be recalled from Section 2.3.2 that patterns confined to the upper or lower fields (Figs 2.16(i) and (j)) are less epileptogenic than when the pattern is confined to the lateral visual field (Figs 2.16(g) and(h)) suggesting some process of integration within a cerebral hemisphere. Illusions show no difference between patterns presented in the upper, lower, and lateral visual fields. This might be because the processes involved in the induction of illusions are more focal and do not spread widely within a cerebral hemisphere. The spread of excitation may be just sufficient to provoke an anomalous excitation of neighbouring neurones within the network, neurones whose activity is responsible for anomalous perceptual effects.

The second difference between the patterns that induce illusions and those that induce epileptiform activity concerns the effects of pattern motion. In Chapter 2 it was shown that patterns that drifted continually towards the centre of gaze were not epileptogenic, whereas those that had similar velocity but repeatedly reversed direction could be highly epileptogenic. This

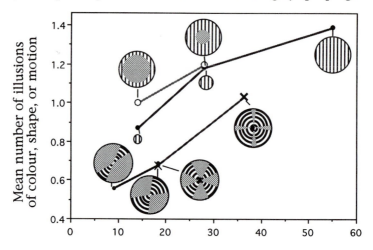

Percentage of visual cortex to which the pattern
projected, Q

Fig. 3.2 The effects of concentric rings and annuli of stripes on perceptual distortions. The size of the pattern of sectored concentric rings can be increased by doubling the sector angles, or the number of sectors. The size of annuli of stripes can be varied by changing the internal or external radius. When size is manipulated in these various ways, the number of illusions seen depends on the area of visual cortex to which the pattern projects. The figures beside each point in the graph represent the pattern schematically. (After Wilkins *et al.* 1980, 1984.)

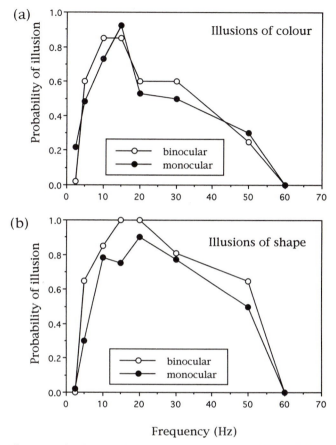

Fig. 3.3 Illusions of colour and shape in response to a diffuse flickering field. The data are from a sample of 15 normal volunteers who reported such illusions when the entire visual field was free of contours and varied in luminance sinusoidally between a minimum of less than 0.01 cd m^{-2} and a maximum of 25 cd m^{-2}. (C. Neary, unpublished data.)

difference does *not* occur for illusions, at least those of colour. Figure 3.4 shows the effects of pattern velocity both on illusions of colour and on epileptiform EEG activity, for two types of pattern movement and for phase reversal. (Illusions of colour were studied on their own because the illusions of form and motion are difficult to discriminate when the pattern is itself moving.) The illusions were most likely when the contour velocity was about 7 deg s^{-1} regardless of its direction, and this was the case when the patterns drifted or vibrated. Seven deg s^{-1} is the contour velocity at which epileptiform activity is most likely in patients with photosensitive epilepsy,

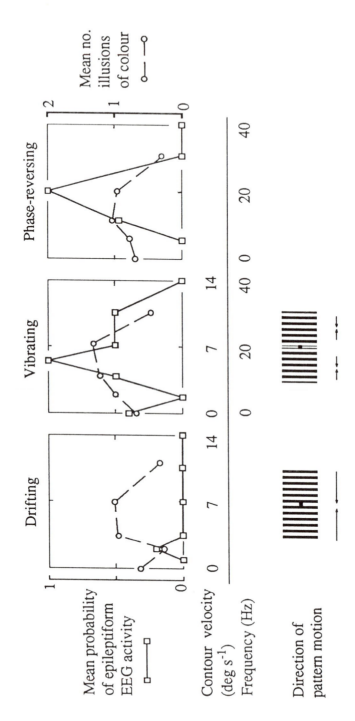

Fig. 3.4 The effects of pattern motion and pattern phase-reversal on illusions and epileptiform EEG activity. The motion was continuous in one direction or repeatedly changed direction, as shown by the arrows.

but only if the pattern is vibrating. If the pattern is drifting, no epileptiform activity occurs.

As has been argued above, many of the illusions, including at least some of colour, may have a common cortical basis. If such an explanation is advanced for the colours seen in drifting or vibrating stripes, the differential effects of pattern motion on illusions and epileptiform activity are easily explained in terms of the role of synchronization. In Chapter 2 it was argued that synchronization of neural activity was necessary at the inception of an epileptiform discharge, and that drifting patterns failed to provide the necessary rhythmic activity. It was argued above that the physiological excitation necessary for illusions is more focal and does not spread widely within a cerebral hemisphere. One might anticipate that it does not spread widely because the cortex is not sufficiently hyperexcitable. The synchronization of large populations of neurones in different cortical areas is not therefore relevant, and so the illusions do not show differential effects of pattern motion.

3.4 Illusions and discomfort

The illusions tend to be associated with discomfort. In various experiments reported by Wilkins *et al.* (1984) observers were asked to give a preference for one of several patterns. The patterns that induced illusions tended not to be preferred, even under conditions in which the effects of bias (range effects: Poulton 1979) were carefully controlled. After prolonged observation some observers reported nausea or a headache. Clearly the patterns can have unfortunate effects not only for patients with epilepsy but for many other people.

3.5 Illusions and headaches

The illusions induced by striped patterns are related to headaches in various ways, as will now be described.

3.5.1 Headache frequency

People who are susceptible to illusions when they observe the pattern in the frontispiece tend to suffer headaches more frequently than those who are not. This relationship has been uncovered in several studies. Subjects were asked to estimate the frequency of their headaches in response to the following question: 'Think of the headaches you have had in the last month, and whether they have been getting more frequent or less frequent. Use this information to help you give your best guess as to how many headaches you have had in the last 12 months.' (Preliminary studies showed that responses to this question correlated well with the number of headaches reported in diaries kept for a one-month period.) The correlation between the number of headaches reported and the number of illusions reported is shown in Fig. 3.5. The correlation might, of course, have occurred for a number of reasons. Some people are more prepared than others to admit to borderline phenomena, be they illusions or headaches, and the correlation could have occurred for this reason. It is therefore interesting that the correlation was negligible when people were asked to report the frequency of events other than headache such as back pain or absent-minded errors. Furthermore, the correlation appeared only when the spatial frequency of the pattern was in

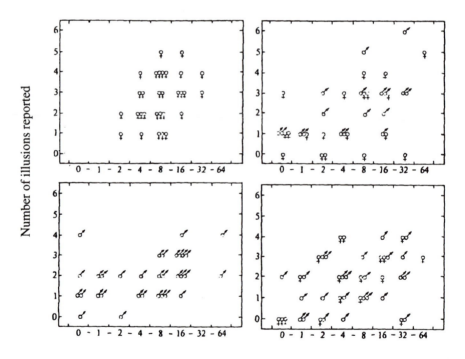

Estimated annual incidence of headaches

Fig. 3.5 The association between the number of illusions seen in patterns of stripes and the number of headaches suffered by the observer. Each panel illustrates data from a different experiment with different subjects and slight variations in procedure. (After Wilkins *et al.* 1984.)

the epileptic range, a finding which is difficult to explain in terms of response bias alone (Wilkins *et al.* 1984).

3.5.2 Time of occurrence

People are more susceptible to illusions on days when they have a headache, and even on the day before. In two studies (Nulty *et al.* 1987; Neary *et al.* in preparation), volunteers were asked to observe a pattern similar to the frontispiece for five seconds, noting the illusions on a check list. They did so every day for at least a month, once in the morning and once in the evening. In the first study the volunteers were people who admitted to chronic worry and in the second, people with severe headaches. In both studies more illusions were reported on days when a headache occurred and in the 24 hours prior to the onset of a headache.

3.5.3 Types of headache

The above studies have uncovered a relationship between the illusions seen in patterns of stripes on the one hand, and visual discomfort, headaches, and headache-proneness on the other. Marcus and Soso (1989) investigated visual discomfort more directly and objectively. They selected 85 hospital staff, many of whom had migraine, and 17 headache patients (who were neurologically normal). They asked each person to look at a set of patterns. Only two patterns in the set had characteristics similar to the frontispiece, the remainder were used as a control. Any objective sign of aversion was noted, such as head withdrawal, deviation of gaze, or grimace with eye-narrowing. None of the control patterns induced such a response. Thirty-five of the 102 subjects clearly found the grating patterns aversive, and 31 (88 per cent) of these had a diagnosis of migraine. Of the 67 who did not show aversion, only 7 (10 per cent) had migraine. Expressing the data a different way, 82 per cent of the 38 subjects with migraine demonstrated an aversion, whereas only 18 per cent of the subjects who suffered non-migrainous headaches did so. The data are summarized in Fig. 3.6. They suggest a strong association between migraine and visual discomfort, but much depends on the definition of migraine.

Marcus and Soso defined migraine by a mixture of four necessary characteristics (history of recurrent headaches, duration 2–72 h, onset before 40 years of age, sufficiently severe as to interrupt routine) together with a set of other contributory characteristics (such as nausea, etc.) from which they compiled a score that had to be exceeded. Their criteria therefore differ slightly from those set out by the International Headache Society (Olesen 1988). The Society has introduced a system of classification of headaches in which *migraine without aura* is a term used to refer to headaches lasting

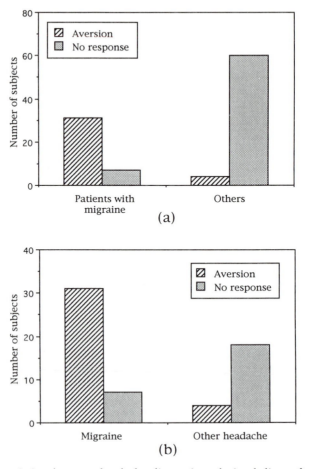

Fig. 3.6 Association between headache diagnosis and visual discomfort (as exemplified by an aversion of gaze): (a) for a sample of headache sufferers and others; (b) for headache sufferers. (After Marcus and Soso 1989.)

4–72 h (untreated or unsuccessfully treated) with pain that has at least two of the following characteristics:

(1) it is confined to one side of the head;

(2) it has a pulsating quality;

(3) it is sufficiently severe as to limit daily activities;

(4) it is aggravated by physical activity.

In addition, at least one of the following associated symptoms must be present during the headache:

(1) nausea with or without vomiting;

(2) an aversion to light (*photophobia*) or to sound (*phonophobia*).

Finally, in order to receive a diagnosis of *migraine without aura*, patients should be free of pain between attacks and should have suffered at least five attacks with the above characteristics. It will be evident that the classification is arbitrary, and that many headaches will be borderline, having some of the characteristics on some occasions and not on others. About 10 per cent of patients with migraine experience an *aura* in addition to the above symptoms of headpain and nausea etc. (Selby and Lance 1960).[1] The aura consists of reversible neurological symptoms such as flashing lights, zigzag lines, partial loss of vision, unilateral numbness, weakness or tingling in the body, difficulty with speech or in finding words. One or more of these symptoms may occur, developing gradually over several minutes, but (by definition) lasting less than an hour.

The visual aura can take a variety of forms and consist of perceptual distortions of space as well as fragmentary loss of vision. The zigzag lines referred to above may begin at the centre of the visual field and then spread outwards on one side. As they spread outwards they usually increase in size and velocity. The changes are what would be expected if the visual phenomena were the result of a disturbance that progressed steadily through the visual cortex at about 3 mm per minute (Richards 1971).

Migraine is distinguished from *tension-type* headache in which the pain is usually of a pressing or tightening quality, of mild or moderate intensity, bilateral, and unaffected by routine physical activity. Nausea is absent, although photophobia or phonophobia may be present.

In practice many people suffer headaches of more than one type and the classificatory criteria can be difficult to apply, particularly where they rely on the patients' memory for details that have been forgotten. Inevitably the distinctions become blurred. Note that photophobia may be present in both migraine and tension-type headaches.

3.5.4 Unilateral illusions

When they keep their eyes on the dot in the centre of the frontispiece most people report that the illusions they see are roughly equally prominent on both sides of the centre. A few, however, report that the illusions are more pronounced on one side. These individuals are more likely than others to experience head pain that is consistently lateralized (Wilkins *et al.* 1984).

---

[1] The proportion will vary with the definition of migraine used, and there is, as yet, no large scale epidemiology based on the definitions of the International Headache Society.

They are therefore also more likely to receive a diagnosis of migraine, given the criteria for migraine outlined in the previous section. Khalil (1991) has shown that in patients who suffer migraine with unilateral visual aura, the side of the aura is almost invariably the side on which the illusions predominate between attacks. It is almost as if the illusions are a 'mini aura', but one that is insufficient to spread. One optometrist known to the author reported that the pattern shown in the frontispiece reliably precipitated his migraine aura, and in two patients reported by Marcus and Soso 'migraine symptoms were induced within several hours of stripe viewing'. Nevertheless, Marcus and Soso (1989) failed to find any difference in susceptibility to stripes among those who suffered migraine with aura, and those whose attacks were without aura. The susceptibility to discomfort from stressful visual stimuli would therefore appear to be just as prominent in people who suffer migraine with aura as in those who experience no aura. Perhaps susceptibility to visual stimuli reflects changes at a very early stage in a chain of pathophysiological events that can culminate in a variety of different manifestations of migraine.

3.6 Underlying pathophysiology

We have seen that illusion susceptibility is increased in migraine. In some people, visual stimulation may provide a triggering factor. There are many such triggering factors, including those that are specific, such as particular foods, and those that are more general, such as stress. In seeking an explanation why, it is helpful to review the two major, and apparently opposing, theories of the aetiology of migraine: the vascular and the neurogenic.

The vascular theory supposes that the disorder is primarily the result of a failure of the mechanisms that regulate the supply of blood to the brain. These may involve the neurotransmitter *serotonin* (also called 5-hydroxytrypamine, or 5-HT for short). Some migraine patients have increased urinary levels of the 5-HT metabolite 5-HIAA (5-hydroxyindoleascetic acid) during an attack. Blood platelet levels of 5-HT fall, and plasma and urinary 5-HT levels rise (Anthony and Lance 1975). Heyck (1969) measured the arterial and venous oxygen content of neck vessels in migraine patients during an attack and found a reduction in the normal differences. He proposed that arterial blood was by-passing the capillaries via shunt vessels (*arteriovenous anastomoses*) and entering directly into the venous system. The existence of arteriovenous shunts in human *dura mater* has subsequently been confirmed, but their relevance to migraine is uncertain. Both the change in 5-HT levels and the shunting may be a consequence of a migraine attack rather than a cause, although a recent drug, *sumatriptan*, that reduces pain during an attack has been shown to reduce the carotid shunt (den Boer *et al.* 1991).

Injection of radioactive xenon (radioisotope ^{133}Xe) into the carotid artery enables measurements of blood flow in the brain to be made during a migraine attack, although with some considerable error ascribed to Compton Scatter (Skyhoj-Olsen and Lassen 1989). In attacks of migraine without aura these measurements seem to suggest little in the way of abnormal activity of the blood vessels within the brain. Migraine with aura does seem to be associated with alterations in regional cerebral blood flow, but even here there is no correlation between the sites of increased and decreased blood flow and the headpain and nausea. The results from one group conflict with those from another (Blau and Drummond 1991). It is not clear whether the site of pain is blood vessels inside the brain or those on the scalp: both may contribute. Only one thing is certain, the notion originally advanced by Wolff (1963) that the aura is due to the constriction of blood vessels, and the pain due to their subsequent dilatation is too simple.

Whether or not the disease process is primarily vascular, it is generally (but not universally) agreed that an attack of migraine is precipitated by neural rather than vascular activity. Many patients have visual aura preceding the onset of migraine, suggesting that the process that triggers the attack originates in the posterior part of the brain. The nature of the zigzag lines of certain aura leave little doubt that, in these circumstances at least, the visual cortex is involved.

Spreading depression is a slow change in brain electrical activity discovered by Leão (1944). It is due to massive depolarization of the neuronal membrane and can be brought about in animals by a variety of cerebral insults. A self-sustaining wave of increased metabolic activity is followed by decreased metabolic activity. Leão himself later suggested that spreading depression might play a part in migraine, as did Milner (1958). In animals, spreading depression initiates a reduction of regional cerebral blood flow of the order of 20–30 per cent which lasts for at least one hour (Lauritzen *et al.* 1982). Slow magnetic field shifts originate in the occipital cortex of migraine patients during the early (*prodromal*) stages of an attack. These resemble the slow changes seen in spreading depression, but there is still controversy whether spreading depression is a phenomenon that occurs in man (Gloor 1986). If migraine is indeed a form of spreading depression, the pain may be triggered in the pain-sensitive fibres in the ventral brain surface by the change of the extracellular microenvironment that results. Attacks could be triggered due to an exaggerated physiological stimulation and this would be consistent with the findings described in the earlier part of this chapter. The similarity between the visual stimuli that provoke seizures and those that give discomfort is of interest in view of the early finding by Van Harreveld and Stamm (1955) that animals will produce spreading depression when they receive visual stimulation, if they have been pretreated with *metrazol* (a drug that increases the likelihood of seizures).

There are abnormalities in patients with migraine not only during the headache, but also between attacks. These are both neural and vascular. There are differences in the EEG responses to visual stimulation (see Winter 1987, for review), and abnormalities in blood flow in the scalp (e.g. Morley and Hunter 1983). It is difficult to know whether these differences are a feature of the disease itself or are caused by minor cerebral damage from repeated attacks perhaps due to an impoverished blood supply (*oligaemia*) (see Olesen 1987). Khalil (1991) has made a contribution to this debate by showing that the ability of a patient to see faint patterns (*contrast sensitivity*; see Section 2.2.3) is impaired to an extent that depends on the duration of the disease rather than simply on age. In migraine with unilateral aura, the decrease is confined to the affected side. Khalil found no relation between disease duration and susceptibility to illusions. This suggests that not all aspects of visual function are equivalently related to disease duration, and further emphasizes the links between illusions and the triggering of headaches.

As we will see in the next chapter, the visual stimuli that induce seizures are those that are neurologically stressful in a large number of different respects. Perhaps the neurological activity in response to these stimuli is exceptionally great and places demands on a vascular system that is compromised.

3.7 Illusions and other bodily differences

There are other bodily differences characterizing individuals susceptible to illusions, as shown by the vulnerability to a virus. Smith *et al.* (1992) included a test of illusion susceptibility in a battery of psychological tests administered to volunteers before and after exposure to various common cold viruses. They presented a pattern similar to the frontispiece and used the checklist described in Section 3.1. Some of the subjects received the virus and some a placebo. Some of those who received the virus developed symptoms of a cold, including headaches, and some did not. Of those who remained symptom-free, some developed an immune reaction and some did not. Before challenge with respiratory syncytial virus, the illusions were more pronounced in the group who subsequently developed symptoms of a cold. This result was obtained in two independent studies. No such effect emerged with corona virus or rhinovirus. Respiratory syncytial virus is common in childhood, commonly resulting in wheeziness (Rooney and Williams 1971), and predisposing to asthma (Sly and Hibbert 1989). We have seen earlier in this chapter how the illusions are related to migraine. It may therefore be significant that children born to women with migraine are more likely to suffer asthma, and the risks of asthma among children born to women who suffer both migraine and asthma/allergies are greater than the risk associated with each individual disease (Chen and Leviton 1990). As we will see in later chapters, many children who have difficulty learning to read report illusions, and many of these children suffer asthma and have migraine in the family. The illusions may reflect a brain state that itself reflects aspects of immune system function.

4   Strong stimulation

Visual discomfort results from the processing of a strong sensory signal. The mechanisms for the pain may resemble those in migraine, but are otherwise quite unclear.

In the two previous chapters we saw that certain visual stimuli may provoke epileptic seizures, headaches, and visual discomfort. It was argued that these adverse effects result from excessive neural activity in those areas of the brain concerned with vision, particularly the visual cortex. In this chapter, the argument is developed. It is shown that the visual stimuli that trigger seizures and anomalous visual effects are physiologically 'strong' stimuli. The stimuli are (1) the easiest to detect at threshold and (2) hardest to ignore when perceiving something else; they also (3) give rise to a large electrical and vascular response in the brain.

4.1 Sensory thresholds

It is common to measure the sensitivity of the human visual system by changing just one particular aspect of a visual stimulus. For example, the contrast of a grating may be reduced until the component bars can only just be seen. It turns out that the contrast at which a grating can just be seen, the *threshold* contrast, depends on the various spatial properties of the grating. One such property is its spatial frequency (i.e. the number of cycles of the grating in one degree subtended at the eye). The spatial frequency at which the threshold is minimal varies with the *field size*, that is, the area of visual field occupied by the grating (see Fig. 4.1). When the grating is large and has low contrast, we are best at detecting it at spatial frequencies close to 2–3 cycle deg^{-1}, provided the luminance is within the photopic range, and provided the observer *fixates* (gazes at) the centre (Campbell and Robson 1968). This is true for gratings with sine-wave and square-wave luminance profiles (Section 2.2). As we saw in Chapters 2 and 3, 3 cycle deg^{-1} is the spatial frequency at which the aversive effects of gratings are most likely, at least when the grating has a large diameter (see Fig. 3.1(c)). In Chapter 2 we saw that the worst spatial frequency depended on viewing position and was lower for gratings presented in the periphery of the visual field, see Fig. 2.18(c). A similar dependence on viewing position obtains with respect to contrast threshold (Robson and Graham 1981).

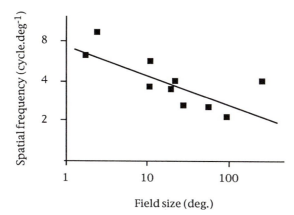

Fig. 4.1 The peak of the contrast sensitivity function as a function of field size. The data are from 10 independent studies, each represented by a single point. Reading from left to right the studies are Blakemore and Campbell (1969); Sjörstrand and Frisen (1977); Hess and Howell (1977), *lower*; Bodis-Wollner and Diamond (1973), *upper*; Regan *et al.* (1977); Plant and Zimmern (unpublished); Derefeldt *et al.* (1979); Beazley *et al.* (1980); Campbell and Robson (1968); Arundale (1978). After Plant *et al.* (1983).

Of course, the contrast threshold at which gratings can be seen depends on many characteristics other than spatial frequency and viewing position. The width of the bars relative to each other is also important. As we saw earlier, the ratio of the width of the bright bar relative to one pattern cycle is referred to as the *duty cycle*. The contrast threshold is lowest when the duty cycle is about 50 per cent, that is when the light and dark bars have the same width. Once again, this is the value at which aversive effects are most likely, see Fig. 3.1(d).

Checkerboard patterns differ from gratings in that contrast varies in two dimensions rather than one. They can have higher contrast thresholds (Kelly 1972) and are generally slightly less aversive, see Fig. 3.1(a).

Campbell and Robson (1968) argued that the visibility of patterns of low contrast reflects the activity of *spatial frequency channels*. The properties of aversive patterns shown in Fig. 3.1 would be such as to maximize the energy in mid-range spatial frequency channels, where the human visual system is most sensitive. The greater susceptibility to patterns with 50 per cent duty cycle (see Section 2.2 and Fig. 3.1) can be interpreted as due to greater energy in the spatial frequency channels to which the visual system is most sensitive. The greater epileptogenic properties of gratings with square-wave luminance profile than those with sinusoidal (Section 2.2) can also be interpreted in these terms. Presumably square-wave gratings result in greater excitation than sine-wave gratings of equivalent contrast because of the harmonics of the square-wave. It is evident that, with respect to the spatial properties of a pattern, the patterns that can most readily be seen at threshold contrast are those which result in discomfort at higher contrasts. As will now be shown, a similar relationship emerges for stimuli that flicker.

A flickering light varies in luminance over time. The proportionate amount by which the light varies, the luminance *modulation*, can be reduced until the flicker is only just perceptible, the modulation threshold. Modulation thresholds depend upon the brightness of a stimulus (its time-averaged luminance) and its size (the angle it subtends at the eye) as well as on its frequency (De Lange 1952). With a large edgeless field the modulation thresholds are lowest for flicker frequencies in the range 12–22 Hz (Kelly 1972). These are the frequencies at which seizures are most likely in those suffering photosensitive epilepsy. In general, most illusions are seen at these frequencies, see Fig. 3.3.

It might be argued that the relationship between threshold sensitivity and aversive effects seen for spatial and for temporal modulation is unsurprising because something cannot have unpleasant effects if it cannot be seen. But note that the aversive effects are obtained well above the threshold at which the stimuli become visible. The thresholds are obtained when some parameter such as contrast is reduced to a minimum whilst a *different* parameter such as spatial frequency or viewing position is varied. At the threshold contrasts at which the visual stimuli can just be seen (less than 0.5 per cent) they are not aversive at all, see Fig. 3.1. Evidently the visual system is most sensitive to these stimuli in a non-pathological as well as a pathological sense.

4.2 Suprathreshold stimuli

Measurement of sensory thresholds gives little indication of the normal physiological response to stronger stimuli that are well above threshold. One way of assessing the response to such suprathreshold stimuli is to measure their effects on other test stimuli that have been optically superimposed. Ruddock and co-workers (Barbur and Ruddock 1980; Grounds *et al.* 1983; Holliday and Ruddock 1983) measured thresholds in a few normal observers for the detection of a small dim circular target moving across a background. The backgrounds were patterned, and could flicker. At high contrasts, patterned backgrounds that had the aversive spatial characteristics shown in Chapter 3 were generally the backgrounds that interfered most with perception, masking the lower contrast target stimulus. The target again became more difficult to see when the background was made to flicker, and when the brightness and frequency were such as would provoke seizures in patients with photosensitive epilepsy. This description does not do justice to the complexity of the threshold functions obtained by Ruddock's group, although in general, aversive stimuli were more effective at masking the probe stimulus.

Chronicle, Wilkins, and Coleston (in preparation) have extended these findings. They measured the luminance at which a stationary letter became visible when superimposed on a square-wave grating. The letter size was a constant ratio of the spatial period of the grating. Two different ratios were used, and the findings were similar for each. When the grating had a spatial frequency of approximately 3 cycle deg^{-1} the letter was most difficult to see, just as in the above experiments, see Fig. 4.2. Chronicle *et al.* also studied the effect of pattern radius when the spatial frequency was 3 cycle deg^{-1}. The larger patterns masked the target letter more effectively than the small patterns, even though the small patterns were themselves quite large enough to cover the letter. When the contrast necessary to see the target was plotted as a function of the proportion of the visual cortex to which the pattern projected (Q), a straight line was obtained, see Fig. 4.3. The linear functions are reminiscent of those in Fig. 3.2 showing the increase in illusions with Q. Using a different probe stimulus, Chronicle *et al.* also studied the effect of

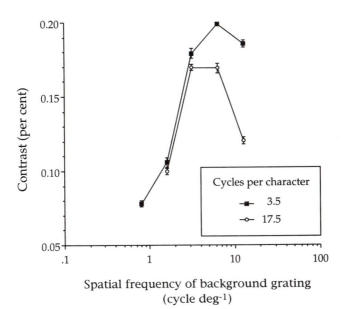

Spatial frequency of background grating
(cycle deg^{-1})

Fig. 4.2 Contrast threshold for a target letter superimposed on a square-wave grating, expressed as a function of the spatial frequency of the grating. Contrast is here defined as $(l_t - l_b)/l_b$ where l_t and l_b are the luminance of the target and background respectively. Bars show standard errors. (After Chronicle *et al.*, in preparation.)

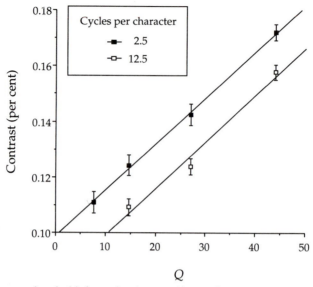

Fig. 4.3 Contrast threshold for a letter superimposed on a square-wave grating, expressed as a function of Q, the percentage of cortex to which the pattern projects. Bars show standard errors. (After Chronicle *et al.*, in preparation.)

the duty cycle of a grating on its capacity to mask superimposed stimuli. The space-averaged luminance of the grating was held constant. The symmetrical function shown in Fig. 4.4 was obtained. Again, the data are consistent with the notion that the greater the physiological excitation induced by a visual stimulus, the greater its interference with the perception of other stimuli, and the more aversive it becomes.

As part of an investigation of the effects of coloured lighting, to be described in Chapter 9, Chronicle *et al.* also showed that the masking of a probe letter was greater in subjects with migraine. This finding is therefore consistent with the greater susceptibility of these subjects to perceptual distortion and visual discomfort, described in Chapter 3.

In the experiments reviewed so far in this chapter, the physiological response to a visual stimulus has been inferred from psychophysical thresholds. We turn now to more direct measurements.

4.3 Aggregate neuronal response

The measurement of *evoked potentials* provides an indication of the way in which a group of neurones act in concert in response to a sensory stimulus. Evoked potentials are the small voltages measurable at the scalp resulting from the electrical activity of the brain in response to a stimulus. Certain cortical neurones increase their firing rate when a visual stimulus is presented, while others are inhibited. Of those that respond to the stimulus, some do so transiently when the stimulus is first presented, others continue to sustain their activity throughout stimulus presentation. Changes in neuronal activity of this kind alter the composite electrical fields that result from the activity of large numbers of neurones. The orientation of these fields with respect to electrodes on the scalp determines how easily the electrical signal can be recorded. The fluctuations in the electrical field reaching the electrode form the *evoked potential*. The evoked potential is therefore a difference signal from a poorly defined set of appropriately oriented neurones, some that fire more strongly and some that reduce their firing rate in response to a change in the sensory stimulus.

Because the voltages are so small it is necessary to average the EEG from many stimulus presentations. The averaging adds only the electrical activity that is time-locked to the stimulus, thus reducing the proportionate contribution from other electrical activity. The evoked potential averaged from several trials usually has a waveform consisting of alternate peaks and troughs each occurring at a different time (latency) after the stimulus.

The amplitude of the waveform is dependent on many things. It is possible to have a large evoked potential from small populations of neurones that fire in such a way that their electrical fields add up, and also to have a small evoked potential from very large populations of neurones whose activity

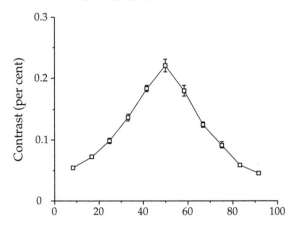

Duty cycle of grating (per cent)

Fig. 4.4 Contrast threshold for a line target superimposed on a square-wave grating, expressed as a function of the duty cycle of the grating. Bars show standard errors. (After Chronicle *et al.*, in preparation.)

is such that the electrical fields cancel each other out. The characteristics of the evoked potential are therefore only an approximate indication of the aggregate neurological response to a stimulus.

Notwithstanding the above limitations, the latency and amplitude of the evoked potential show systematic relationships to the characteristics of a visual stimulus, and some of these are consistent from one individual to another.

Campbell and Maffei (1974) and Plant *et al.* (1983) studied the potential evoked by sine-wave gratings. The gratings appeared and disappeared repeatedly, or repeatedly reversed their phase (white bars changing to black, black to white). The amplitudes of the potentials depended on the particular waveforms measured, and on the nature of the change in the pattern that evoked them. The amplitude of the response increased with the size of the pattern (field size). For a 10-degree pattern the maximum amplitude occurred with spatial frequencies close to 3 cycle deg^{-1}, as can be seen from Fig. 4.5. The highest amplitude evoked potential occurred at spatial frequencies similar to those at which contrast sensitivity was greatest. Figure 3.1(c) shows that, for a similarly sized square-wave grating, 3 cycle deg^{-1} is the spatial frequency at which aversive effects are most likely.

The visual evoked potential in response to a rapidly repeating stimulus, such as a flickering light, requires different techniques for assessment because

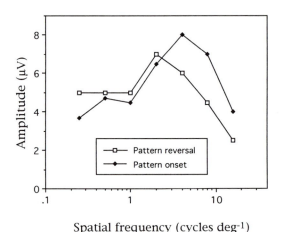

Spatial frequency (cycles deg^{-1})

Fig. 4.5 The amplitude of the first positive peak of the potential evoked by the onset or phase-reversal of a grating with sine-wave luminance profile, radius 10 deg, expressed as a function of the spatial frequency of the grating. (After Plant *et al.* 1983.)

the later components of the response to one flash are superimposed on the earlier components of the response to the next. Instead of averaging the EEG, Fourier analysis is often used to assess the power at various frequencies (Spekreijse *et al.* 1977). Figure 4.6 shows the amplitude of the fundamental Fourier component (the component at the frequency of the stimulating light). In this subject it peaks at a frequency close to that at which flickering light is most epileptogenic, cf. Fig. 2.3.

We have already seen in Chapter 3 that the EEG in people with migraine differs from that of normals. People who are prone to headaches show abnormally large evoked potentials in response to flicker at frequencies that are maximally epileptogenic: those close to 20 Hz (see Winter 1987, for review). They can sometimes also show non-specific EEG changes resembling epileptiform EEG activity (Goldensohn 1976).

The association between the stimuli that give the largest evoked potentials and those that have aversive effects is not perfect. Patterns that vary in more than one orientation, such as chequerboards, can often elicit slightly higher amplitude evoked potentials than stripes, depending on the size of the checks. Chequerboard stimuli are generally slightly less likely to provoke discomfort, see Chapters 2 and 3.

The evidence for a large aggregate neural response at frequencies close to those that are maximally epileptogenic is not confined to electrophysiology.

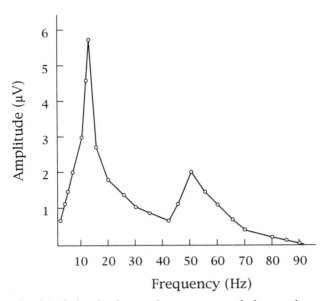

Fig. 4.6 Amplitude of the fundamental component of the steady-state evoked potential in response to a diffuse flickering field. (After Spekreijse *et al.* 1977.)

Fox and Raichle (1984) measured regional cerebral blood flow in the human brain using positron emission tomography. They presented 30 red lights arranged in a 5 × 6 grid subtending 45 deg. The display flashed at rates of 1.0, 3.9, 7.8, 15.5, 33.1, and 61 Hz. The flicker caused a selective increase in regional cerebral blood flow in the occipital cortex, and the increase depended on frequency according to a curvilinear function shown in Fig. 4.7. The frequency at which the maximum increase occurred cannot be determined precisely from these data, given the spacing of points and the standard deviation at each point, but it would appear to be between 7.8 and 30 Hz, close to the frequency range at which flicker is maximally epileptogenic.

From the evidence discussed so far, it appears that the stimuli that induce visual discomfort are those that cause intense and widespread activation of the visual cortex and that they do so because the visual system is designed to be maximally sensitive to the visual input provided by those stimuli. As we have seen in Chapter 2, when a vertical grating and a horizontal grating are optically superimposed, the plaid pattern that results is less epileptogenic than either of its individual vertical and horizontal components. One might have expected the plaid pattern to be more epileptogenic because it has twice

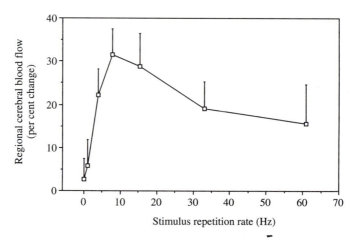

Fig. 4.7 Regional cerebral blood flow (rCBF) measured by positron emission tomography and expressed as a percent change from an initial scan with no visual stimulation. Measurements were made from an occipital brain region of constant area. The position of the area remained identical for all scans from an individual subject, but was chosen to be close to the region at which that individual showed the greatest change. The data show the average and standard deviation of nine subjects (eight for 1 Hz and 61 Hz). (After Fox and Raichle 1984.)

as much energy as either single grating from which it is composed. On the other hand, Morrone *et al.* (1982) recorded electrical activity from simple and complex cells in the striate cortex and showed that the response to gratings was reduced when orthogonal gratings were optically superimposed, attributing the reduction to intracortinal inhibition. Whatever the mechanism for the reduction, their finding shows that the reduced aversive response to plaid patterns is consistent with the idea that the aversion results from an intense and widespread activation of the visual cortex.

A simple and uncontroversial idea has emerged in this chapter: discomfort arises from strong physiological stimulation to which the visual system is most sensitive. Other more speculative ideas are developed in Chapter 10.

5 Reading

Reading can provoke 'pattern-glare', resulting in illusions, eye-strain, head-aches, and seizures. It does so because the successive lines of printed text resemble a pattern of stripes, and the 'stripes' have spatial characteristics within the critical range. The striped properties vary considerably from one text to another and depend in part on the horizontal spacing of the words relative to the vertical spacing of the lines. Most text can be made clearer and easier to read by covering the lines that are not being read. It may be possible to change the characteristics of conventional text slightly and improve clarity without increasing costs.

In Chapter 2 we described how certain patterns of stripes can induce seizures in patients with photosensitive epilepsy, and in Chapter 3 we showed that these same patterns are judged unpleasant by people who do not have epilepsy, especially those who suffer headaches and eye-strain. The patterns are not only unpleasant to look at, they induce a variety of anomalous visual effects, effects to which those with headache and eye-strain are particularly susceptible. In this chapter it is shown that text can have aversive characteristics and that these relate less to the design of the typeface than to the spacing of characters on the page.

It is only when they have certain very specific spatial characteristics that patterns become aversive and induce anomalous visual effects and unpleasant neurological sequelae. As described in Chapters 2 and 3, the worst patterns are those of black and white stripes, particularly

(1) when the pattern is large;

(2) when each stripe subtends about 10 min of arc at the eye (i.e. the spatial frequency of the pattern is about 3 cycle deg^{-1};

(3) when the stripes have an even width and spacing (a duty cycle close to 50 per cent); and

(4) when the stripes are bright and strongly contrasting.

The effects of these pattern characteristics are shown in Fig. 3.1. The frontispiece of this book provides an example of an aversive pattern with spatial characteristics for which illusions and seizures are likely. **Do not look at the frontispiece if you have epilepsy or migraine.**

5.1 Text as a striped pattern

The successive lines of text form a pattern rather like that of stripes. If you look at the text in Fig. 5.1 and almost close your eyes so that you can no longer see detail, the stripes will become more apparent. You may find the text in Fig. 5.1 more difficult to read than the identical material on this page, and that it becomes clearer when the lines above and below those you are reading are covered up. The text in Fig. 5.1 has been altered so that the spacing of lines and letters increases the effect of the stripes, as will be described.

5.2 Measuring the 'stripes' of text

The angular size of the grating-like pattern that text provides is determined by the size of the page (less the margins) and the distance from which the text is read. The reading distance and the interline spacing combine to determine the spatial frequency of the grating (the number of spatial cycles of the pattern in one degree of angle subtended at the eye). The ascenders and descenders of letters contribute little to the mean line density profile of a line of text (Wilkins and Nimmo-Smith 1987). If, for the sake of simplicity the ascenders and descenders are ignored, the width of the stripes depends on the height of the central body of the letters, or *x-height*, and the *x*-height and interline spacing combine to provide an estimate of the ratio of bar width to bar separation (duty cycle) of the grating. The contrast of the grating is determined by the contrast of the ink on the paper and the width and spacing of the letter strokes and can be estimated from the space-averaged reflectance of a line of text, and measured using simple photometric methods (Wilkins and Nimmo-Smith 1987).

The horizontal bars in Fig. 3.1 show, for typical text, the range of values of each pattern characteristic. These values were obtained in a study by Wilkins and Nimmo-Smith (1987) who asked volunteers to select books from their personal libraries, choosing those with 'clear' and 'less clear' text. They were asked to position the book at a comfortable reading distance and measure the distance from their eyes to the page. In the first of two studies the volunteers were students aged 18–25. In the second study, other adults aged 19–63 took part.

Table 5.1 gives the average values of reading distance, interline spacing, *x*-height, and page width for the two samples of books. Figure 5.2 shows the way in which these measurements were obtained. They were used to calculate the subtense, spatial frequency, and duty cycle of the 'grating' formed by text, and the values of these variables are shown in Fig. 3.1

5.1 Text as a striped pattern

The successive lines of text form a pattern rather like that of stripes. If you look at the text in Figure 5.1 and almost close your eyes so that you can no longer see detail, the stripes will become more apparent. You may find the text in Figure 5.1 more difficult to read than the identical material on this page, and that it becomes clearer when the lines above and below those you are reading are covered up. The text in Figure 5.1 has been altered so that the spacing of lines and letters increases the effect of the stripes, as will be described.

5.2. Measuring the "stripes" of text

The angular size of the grating-like pattern that text provides is determined by the size of the page (less the margins) and the distance from which the text is read. The reading distance and the interline spacing combine to determine the spatial frequency of the grating (the number of spatial cycles of the pattern in one degree of angle subtended at the eye). The ascenders and descenders of letters contribute little to the mean line density profile of a line of text (Wilkins and Nimmo-Smith, 1987). If, for the sake of simplicity the ascenders and descenders are ignored, the width of the stripes depends on the height of the central body of the letters, or *x-height*, and the x-height and interline spacing combine to provide an estimate of the ratio of bar width to bar separation (duty cycle) of the grating. The contrast of the grating is determined by the contrast of the ink on the paper and the width and spacing of the letter strokes and can be estimated from the space-averaged reflectance of a line of text, and measured using simple photometric methods (Wilkins and Nimmo-Smith, 1987). The horizontal bars in Figure 3.1 show, for typical text, the range of values of each pattern characteristic. These values were obtained in a study by Wilkins and Nimmo-Smith (1987) who asked volunteers to select books from their personal libraries, choosing those with "clear" and "less clear" text. They were asked to position the book at a comfortable reading distance and measure the distance from their eyes to the page. In the first of two studies the volunteers were students aged 18-25. In the second study, other adults aged 19-63 took part. Table 5.1 gives the average values of reading distance, interline spacing, x-height, and page width for the two samples of books. Figure 5.2 shows the way in which these measurements were obtained. They were used to calculate the subtense, spatial frequency and duty cycle of the "grating" formed by text, and the values of these variables are shown in Figure 3.1

Fig. 5.1 The text on this page is set in such a way as to maximize the probability of seeing illusions. If you look at a letter in the centre of the page for a short while the lines may start to shimmer, and a faint rhomboid lattice may appear. Compare with the text on the previous page.

Table 5.1 Spatial characteristics for samples of 'clear' and 'less clear' text selected by undergraduate students and by other volunteers aged 31–74 (after Wilkins and Nimmo-Smith 1987).

Variable	Mean value of variable				Variance in clarity judgements explained (per cent)	
	'Clear' text		'Less clear' text			
	Students	Others	Students	Others	Students	Others
Reading distance (mm)	345	402	272	339	29.2	30.3
Page height (mm)	165	–	164	–	0.2	–
Page width (mm)	102	–	97	–	2.7	–
x-height (mm)	1.64	1.78	1.47	1.52	26.9	32.5
Interline spacing (mm)	4.38	4.37	3.78	3.41	33.7	37.7
Minimal subtense (deg)	17		20			
Spatial frequency (cycle deg^{-1})	1.4	1.6	1.3	1.7		
Duty cycle (%)	37	41	39	45		
Interletter spacing (mm)	0.30	0.28	0.34	0.30	9.4	3.4
Paper used per character (mm^2)	7.26	8.29	5.59	5.51	6.6	30.3

and in Table 5.1. Note that although the 'less clear' text has lines that are more closely spaced, readers hold their heads closer to the page. This has the effect of reducing the spatial frequency, keeping it away from the maximally noxious values. It is perhaps worth noting that such adjustment of reading materials may be more difficult when text is presented on a visual display.

The contrast of the 'stripes' was more difficult to measure, since each stripe comprises the characters and the spaces between them. To estimate the average contrast of a 'stripe', an optic fibre with a slit 100 mm wide and 1 mm high was used to direct light at a line of text and to measure the light reflected back from the page. When the device was moved down the page the reflectance varied as shown in Fig. 5.3. Note that the ascenders and descenders of the letters contributed little to the shape of the waveform.

The difference between the maximum and minimum reflectance was used to estimate the contrast of a line of text for identical passages of text printed in different founts. Within the range of samples measured the fount had a greater effect on contrast than variables such as the contrast of the ink on

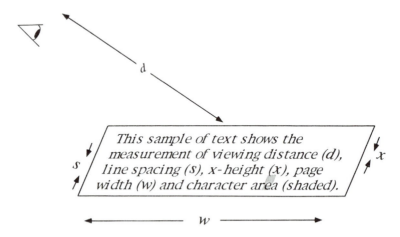

This sample of text shows the measurement of viewing distance (d), line spacing (s), x-height (x), page width (w) and character area (shaded).

Fig. 5.2 Measurements of printed text used to estimate the values of various spatial characteristics, showing the height of the letters or *x-height* (*x*), the spacing from one line to the next (*s*), and the width of the line (*w*). Observers were asked to position the book at a comfortable reading position and to measure the distance from their eye to the page (*d*). The angular size (subtense) of the pattern was estimated as 2arctan(*w*/2*d*), a conservative estimate since most text is usually taller than it is wide. The spatial frequency was calculated as arctan (*s*/*d*), and the duty cycle as (*s*−*x*)/*s*×100 per cent. The cost of printing depends partly on the average area of paper used per character, which is the product of the spacing between the lines and the average horizontal distance from one character to the next. The latter was calculated from the mean number of letters in three successive complete lines (*n*). The area of paper used per character, *s.w*/*n*, is shown by the shaded rectangle. (After Wilkins and Nimmo-Smith 1987.)

the page. As can be seen from Fig. 5.4, the contrasts all lie in the range 14–22 per cent, and are therefore sufficient to provoke illusions, see Fig. 3.1.[1] Notice also that the slope of the contrast function in Fig. 3.1 is such that any differences between founts are unlikely to have a large influence on the aversive effects.

---

[1] These estimates are conservative because they include the mirror-like reflections from the page.

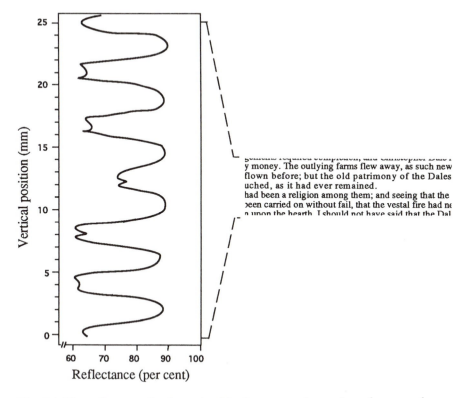

The inset text reads:

> y money. The outlying farms flew away, as such new
> flown before; but the old patrimony of the Dales
> uched, as it had ever remained.
> had been a religion among them; and seeing that the
> been carried on without fail, that the vestal fire had ne
> n upon the hearth. I should not have said that the Dal

Fig. 5.3 The reflectance (horizontal-axis) of a rectangular section of a page of text. The text is shown in the inset. Measurements of reflectance were made from a section of page measuring 100 mm wide by 1 mm high by a device that moved in a vertical direction. The measurements were made at an angle of reflection similar to the angle of incidence and therefore included contribution from mirror-like reflections from the paper. The paper had a matt surface, and so the contribution will have been small. The measurements should nevertheless be taken as conservative estimates of contrast.

5.3 Extending the measurements to two dimensions

Text is a two-dimensional pattern and the stripe-like quality depends on the variation in character density within a line, and the extent to which such variations change from one line to another, as will now be shown.

Consider the two samples of text shown in Fig. 5.5. Both have similar line spacing and character spacing, but in the sample on the left the spaces between neighbouring words are rather small.

Figure 3.1 shows that spatial frequencies in the range 1–8 cycle deg^{-1}

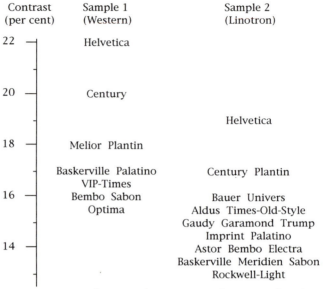

Fig. 5.4 The mean contrasts of rectangular segments of two samples of text printed in a range of founts. The position of the fount name indicates the contrast.

are most likely to be harmful, at least for gratings with sharp edges, or more correctly, those with a square-wave luminance profile. (The narrow spatial tuning of the function suggests that the higher frequency harmonics of the square-wave gratings have only a small effect.) Watt and Wilkins (unpublished observations) filtered samples of text so that only these mid-range spatial frequencies were visible, see Fig. 5.5. They used an electronic camera to convert an image of the text to an array of light intensity measurements. The image was then filtered by a mathematical process known as convolution. Each point or pixel in the image was smoothed by substituting it with a 'blob-like' shape, the height of which depended on the light intensity of that pixel, see Fig. 5.6. The shape has the advantage that the space-averaged luminance remains unaltered. This is because the volume in the peak of the 'Mexican hat' equals the volume in the brim.

The filtering that the convolution performed can be likened to defocusing the original camera image, the degree of 'defocus' depending on the standard deviation of the filter: the width of the 'hat'. The process is mathematically similar to that of removing high spatial frequency components, although the end result is more easily visualized than in a two-dimensional Fourier transform.

Figures 5.5(b) and (c) show the filtered images. In Figure 5.5(c) the standard deviation of the filter is twice as large as in 5.5(b), in other words more of the details (high spatial frequencies) have been removed. Note that the sample on the left is striped and remains so for a wide range of filter settings. In the sample of text on the left the words in a line easily blur together to form a stripe, whereas in the sample on the right the words tend to remain separate. As the standard deviation of the filter is increased, increasing the blur, the words in the sample on the right tend to coalesce with those on lines above and below as much as with those on the same line. In Figs 5.5(d) and (e) the contrast of the filtered image has been exaggerated by setting all luminance values below the mean to black and those above to white. This serves to make the stripes more visible. Those readers who are susceptible to the effects of stripes may see illusions in the patterns on the left, but are less likely to do so in the patterns on the right which have shorter line segments (cf. Fig. 3.1(a)). The text on the right may appear easier to read. For further examples of the effects of filtering see Watt *et al.* (1990).

It has now been shown that text is theoretically appropriate for the induction of illusions, eye-strain, headaches, and seizures. In the sections which follow it is shown that text does indeed provoke these unfortunate effects in people who are visually sensitive: some of those who suffer photophobia or photosensitive epilepsy. The anomalous visual effects and eye-strain are considered first. The evidence concerning seizures is discussed later.

5.4 Anomalous visual effects, eye-strain, and text clarity

Wilkins and Nimmo-Smith (1987) asked normal observers to look at a particular letter in the centre of a page of text for 30 s. Various anomalous visual effects were reported, covering the range of illusions commonly seen in striped patterns, and including a lattice of faint rhomboid shapes: an illusion sometimes reported after prolonged observation of a striped pattern. When text with a larger typeface was used, so that the spatial frequency of the grating was reduced, the size of the rhomboid lattice increased in just the same way as when the spatial frequency of a grating is reduced.

The text in Fig. 5.1 has been typeset in such a way as to render illusions likely. The height of the central body of the letters (*x*-height) has been reduced so that at a typical reading distance of 0.4 m it subtends 10 min of arc at the eye; the lines of text have been separated by spaces of similar height so that the duty cycle of the 'grating' is close to 50 per cent; the contrast of the lines has been increased by reducing the spaces between adjacent letters and words. The spatial characteristics formed by the text are close to those for which illusions are maximally likely. When you look at the paragraph in a strong light the lines may seem to shimmer. If you gaze at a letter in the

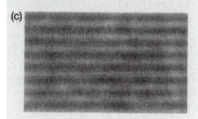

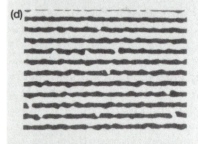
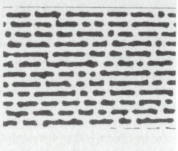

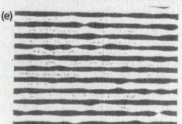
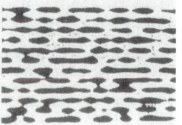

a strong light the lines may seem to shimmer. If you gaze at a letter in the centre of the page for a while, a faint rhomboid lattice may appear. Compare the illusions you see in this paragraph with those seen in the grating in the frontispiece. They will be less intense but are probably similar in nature.

The samples of text shown in Fig. 5.5 were selected by a 41 year old woman who was unable to read for more than about 20 min before she suffered disorientation (which she described as feeling 'disconcerted'). She selected the sample on the left of Fig. 5.5(a) as being particularly difficult to read; the other sample gave her no problems.

The degree to which the lines of text form stripes when blurred in this way depends in part on the relationship between the horizontal spacing between words and the vertical spacing between lines. Figure 5.7 shows these variables for samples of text selected as 'clear' or 'less clear' by undergraduates. As can be seen, 'clear' text tends to have larger spaces between the words and between the lines.

It is perhaps worth noting that the above data were obtained using books that were, for the most part, set in hot metal type. With the advent of electronic typography, text is often set using the default parameters of desk-top publishing software. The default settings of one such software package produce text that has spacing parameters well outside the scatter shown in Fig. 5.7. Further, the new printing methods often result in a greater deposition of ink, enhancing contrast. Contrast is further enhanced by the brightening agents that are now added to paper. These are fluorescent substances that convert ultraviolet light to visible light, making the paper 'whiter-than-white'. All these developments may therefore act to increase the incidence of visual discomfort from reading.

5.5 Preventing eye-strain, headaches, and seizures

In 1897 Prentice described a device which he christened the *Typoscope* and which consisted simply of a card in which was cut a rectangular slot sufficient

---

Fig. 5.5 (left) (a) Two examples of printed text. Both have similar line spacing and character spacing, and yet the sample on the left seems more 'stripey' in some indefinite way. The samples were selected by a 41 year old woman with an inability to read for periods of more than about 20 min without eye-strain and feelings of being 'disconcerted'. She selected the sample on the left as being particularly difficult to read; the sample on the right gave her no problems. In (b) and (c) the samples of text above have been filtered by convolution with a Mexican hat filter, which has the effect of removing the high spatial frequency components. In (c) the filter has a standard deviation twice that in (b). In (d) and (e) the contrast of the filtered images has been exaggerated to make the stripes more apparent.

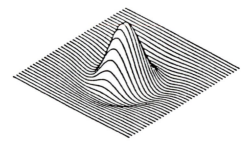

Fig. 5.6 The shape of a Mexican hat filter. The height of the curve represents the contrast of the image at that point, and the hat shape shows the manner in which contrast varies with spatial extent. The filtering in Fig. 5.5 has been achieved by replacing every point (*pixel*) in the image with a blob of contrast shown by Fig. 5.6, the relative height of the peak of the 'hat' is dependent on the contrast of the pixel.

to reveal one line of text when the card was placed on the page of a book (see Mehr 1969). The front surface of the card was matt black and was thought to reduce the effects of scattered light in patients with cataract and those with *amblyopia* (lazy eye) who wore lenses with strong magnification. The device has been re-invented (and different versions patented) several times since then, see Fig. 5.8.

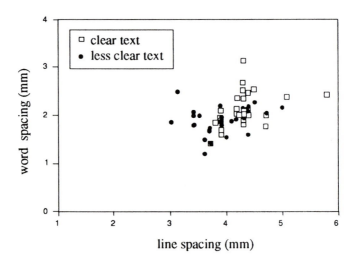

Fig. 5.7 Line spacing and word spacing of samples of text selected by undergraduates as 'clear' (open points) and 'less clear' (filled points).

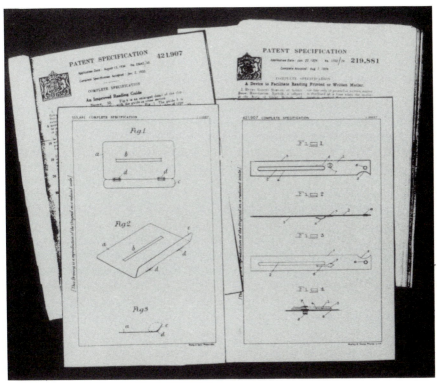

Fig. 5.8 The Prentice Typoscope in two reincarnations.

A reading mask such as the above reduces the effects of the striped pattern by covering the unnecessary stripes. In a study by Wilkins and Nimmo-Smith (1984) about 70 per cent of normal observers noticed that the text in the 'window' of such a mask appeared clearer. The observers who noticed the improvement in clarity tended to be those who reported many illusions in a pattern of striped lines similar to the frontispiece. In the same study about one third of a sample of people who suffered eye-strain or headaches from reading reported that a reading mask was of sufficient benefit to be worth the nuisance of using it. No benefits were reported from placebo aids that did not restrict the lines. These studies helped with the design of an inexpensive reading aid.[2] The device consists simply of two rectangular pieces of grey matt translucent plastic joined along one shorter edge by a

---

[2] The reading aid is now marketed as the *Cambridge Easy Reader* by Engineering and Design Plastics, 84 High Street, Cherry Hinton, Cambridge, UK.

A reading mask reduces the effects of the striped pattern by covering the stripes above and below those being read. This figure shows two identical passages of text, one covered by a reading mask. Compare the clarity of the text in the "window" with that of the identical passage in the unobscured passage below (marked by a vertical bar in the margin). In a study by Wilkins and Nimmo-Smith (1984) about 70% of normal observers reported that the text in the "window" of such a mask appeared clearer. The observers who reported the improvement in clarity tended to report more illusions in a pattern of striped lines than observers who reported no such improvement. In the same study about one third of a sample of people who suffered eye- strain or headaches from reading reported that a reading mask was of sufficient benefit to be worth the nuisance of using it. No benefits were reported from aids that did not cover the lines both above and below those being read. These studies helped with the design of a reading aid which is now marketed as the "Cambridge Easy Reader" by Engineering and Design Plastics, 84 High Street, Cherry Hinton, Cambridge.

A reading mask reduces the effects of the striped pattern by covering the stripes above and below those being read. This figure shows two identical passages of text, one covered by a reading mask. Compare the clarity of the text in the "window" with that of the identical passage in the unobscured passage below (marked by a vertical bar in the margin). In a study by Wilkins and Nimmo-Smith (1984) about 70% of normal observers reported that the text in the "window" of such a mask appeared clearer. The observers who reported the improvement in clarity tended to report more illusions in a pattern of striped lines than observers who reported no such improvement. In the same study about one third of a sample of people who suffered eye- strain or headaches from reading reported that a reading mask was of sufficient benefit to be worth the nuisance of using it. No benefits were reported from aids that did not cover the lines both above and below those being read. These studies helped with the design of a reading aid which is now marketed as the "Cambridge Easy Reader" by Engineering and Design Plastics, 84 High Street, Cherry Hinton, Cambridge.

Fig. 5.9 (a) An illustration of the visual effects of a reading mask. For many observers the text in the window will appear clearer than the identical text in the unmasked paragraph below (marked with a vertical line in the margin). (b) The Cambridge Easy Reader in use.

magnetic slide. Text is viewed in the gap between the plastic rectangles. For an illustration of the visual effect, see Fig. 5.9(a).

Wilkins and Lindsay (1985) reported that the reading aid reduced liability to seizures in patients with epileptic pattern sensitivity. The EEG was recorded during periods of rest, and also during randomly interleaved periods when the patient read a book in the usual way, and when the book was read using the reading mask. The mask darkened and blurred the lines of text above and below those being read, and was adjusted so that it left three lines unobscured. Table 5.2 shows the rate of epileptiform EEG discharges during the three conditions, for the two patients reported by Wilkins and Lindsay and for a third patient subsequently recorded by Darby (personal communication). The incidence of epileptiform discharges was significantly increased by reading, and significantly reduced by the use of the reading mask.

5.6 Improving text without increasing costs

In Sections 5.1–5.3 it has been shown that the pattern from text can provoke illusions, headaches, eye-strain, and even seizures in those who are

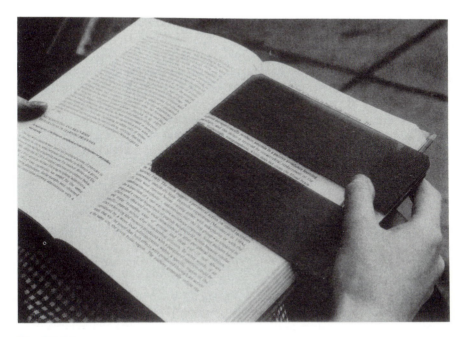

Fig. 5.9 (b)

Table 5.2 Incidence of epileptiform EEG activity (discharges/minute) in three patients with photosensitive epilepsy and pattern sensitivity. The EEG was recorded whilst the patients were at rest and when they read a book with and without a mask that darkened and blurred the lines of text above and below those being read.

	Patient MN	Patient IJ	Patient RB
At rest	0.70	0.00	Not tested
Reading without mask	1.48	2.67	8.52
Reading with mask	0.73	0.58	2.50

After Wilkins and Lindsay (1985) and including further data from RB recorded by Mrs C.E. Darby.

susceptible. The pattern can be reduced by covering irrelevant lines with a reading mask, but according to the theory outlined in Chapter 4, the mask should not be necessary: it should be possible to reduce the effects of the pattern in other ways. One obvious way is to increase the spacing between the lines. As can be seen from Fig. 3.1, this has two effects: it increases the duty cycle and decreases the spatial frequency of the 'grating'. Both changes are in a direction appropriate for a reduction in the adverse effects of the pattern. The clarity of text has long been known to depend upon the spacing of the lines (see, for example, Tinker 1963), and this might be one reason why.

Increasing the spacing of the lines is likely to increase the costs of publishing, because these costs depend partly on the amount of paper used. Can line spacing be increased without increasing costs?

The amount of paper used depends in part on the average area of paper occupied by a character. The average area is the product of the separation of the lines and the mean horizontal distance from one character to the next. As noted earlier, Wilkins and Nimmo-Smith (1987) asked volunteers to select books from their own libraries that had 'clear' or 'less clear' print. They showed that subjects' judgements of clarity were strongly associated with the spacing between the lines, but not so strongly associated with the area of paper used per character. In the two studies, interline spacing accounted for 33.7 per cent and 37.7 per cent of the variance associated with judgements of clarity, see Table 5.1. The average area occupied by a letter explained 6.6 and 30.3 per cent respectively (the difference in the variance explained presumably reflects the relative homogeneity of the typography of books selected by the students). In other words there were books with text judged as 'clear' that cost no more to print than books with text judged as 'less clear'. Evidently printing convention does not specify the spatial characteristics of text appropriately for the maximization of 'clarity' at a given cost.

It should therefore be possible, at least in principle, to improve the clarity of text without making it more expensive. One way of doing so might be to increase the spacing between lines whilst reducing the average spacing between characters. Both these changes would only need to be extremely slight, and both the line spacing and character spacing could remain within the limits set by conventional typographic practice. It would be important to ensure that the decrease in the average horizontal spacing between characters occurred within words, and maintained an appropriate relationship between horizontal word spacing and vertical line spacing. Little experimental work has been undertaken to investigate the effects of these parameters on text clarity, although that which has been done suggests an insignificant effect (Reynolds 1979).

It is worth emphasizing that these suggestions for improvements to printed text are based only on theoretical considerations, and have yet to be put to empirical test. However, an unpublished pilot study by Sheppard and Wilkins has suggested that improvements in clarity may be very much a matter of individual preference. Two groups were selected, one with frequent eye-strain and another with none. Samples of text were prepared with small, medium, or large vertical spacing between the lines, and with small, medium, or large horizontal spacing between the words. The 'medium' spacing parameters were the default values for Aldus *PageMaker*® version 3.1 and the 'small' and 'large' parameters differed by ±10 per cent. The three levels of vertical spacing and the three levels of horizontal spacing provided nine samples of text which were given to subjects in the two groups to rank in order of clarity. The judgements of clarity were more consistent for the group reporting eye-strain, and line spacing had a large effect, with the largest spacing being ranked as clearest. Subjects in the symptom-free group were less consistent. Although they ranked the 'medium' line spacing as clearest, there was little difference between the 'medium' and 'large' line spacing. For both groups, horizontal word spacing had relatively little effect.

We have seen that the typographic layout of text may influence the perception of clarity, and the comfort of reading. But typographic changes that influence comfort are unlikely to affect reading performance, except perhaps indirectly and in the long term. Even in patients with visual reading epilepsy, seizures usually occur only after about 20 min of reading. Nevertheless Poulton (1959, 1960, 1965) studied the effects of typography on comprehension and reported small effects.

5.7 Alternative explanations

The findings described in this chapter have been interpreted from a theoretical position adopted in Chapters 2, 3, and 4. This theory provides a coherent explanation of all the data. Nevertheless some of the findings may also be understood from other viewpoints, in particular those relating to the control of eye movements.

When the eyes move from one point of regard to another they do so in a series of high-velocity jerks known as saccades. Findlay (1982) and Ottes *et al.* (1984) asked observers to make an eye movement to one of two spots, both of which could easily be seen in the periphery of vision. When the spots were close together, the eyes landed at a point in space between the two spots, and then made a subsequent small corrective movement towards the appropriate target. It was difficult, if not impossible, for subjects to learn to move their eyes directly to one of the targets, even though they could distinguish them in peripheral vision before they began the eye movement. It was as if the part of the visual system controlling the first fast movement was unable to distinguish the two spots, but used instead some more global representation. Text in which the words coalesce to form stripes in the mid-range spatial frequencies (e.g. the text on the left in Fig. 5.5) might place greater computational demands on the saccadic system, see O'Regan (in press) for review. As we will see in Chapter 7, the effects of typographic layout may play an even greater role when the control of eye movements is compromised by flicker.

6 Lighting

Most electric lighting pulsates in brightness twice with each cycle of the alternating electricity supply. The pulsations are too rapid ordinarily to be seen as flicker but they affect the firing of visual neurones. Fluorescent lighting pulsates more than incandescent lighting and the pulsation is usually greatest at the blue end of the spectrum. This pulsation may be responsible for more than half the headaches and eye-strain suffered by office workers. Glasses that absorb blue light can reduce the pulsation reaching the eye by about one third and there are initial indications that they help prevent headaches in children with migraine.

In this chapter it is shown that artificial lighting gives rise to visual discomfort due to imperceptible but continuous variation in luminous intensity.

6.1 Characteristics of electric lighting

Most electric lamps produce light in one of two ways – by heating a wire conductor to white heat (incandescent lamps) or by causing a gas to ionize (gas discharge lamps). The lamps are usually powered from an alternating current supply and as a result the light from the lamps varies continuously in brightness, pulsating at a frequency related to that of the electricity supply.

The filament lamp was the earliest form of electric light and it is still the most popular form of lighting in domestic use. The light is *incandescent* (literally, glowing) and is generated when a current is passed through a wire filament. The filament glows white-hot but is prevented from burning by a gas enclosed in a glass bulb. The current from an AC electricity supply varies sinusoidally, increasing in one direction, then decreasing again before reversing direction and increasing and decreasing once more. The white-hot wire is heated regardless of the direction of the current passing thought it, so that the variation in light has a frequency twice that of the supply. The hot wire takes time to cool and so continues to emit light during the phase in the AC supply when the current is low (the lamp exhibits *thermal inertia*). The extent to which the light varies over time differs from one lamp to another, depending partly on the thickness of the wire filament. The variation in light output as a function of time is sinusoidal, see Fig. 6.1.

A fluorescent lamp is lit by a current passed between two heated wires, one

A fluorescent lamp is lit by a current passed between two heated wires, one at each end of a long glass tube containing a gas, usually mercury vapour at low pressure. The gas is caused to ionize by the voltage across the ends of the tube and a discharge (similar to lightning) results. The radiation from the discharge is mainly in the ultraviolet and short-wavelength (blue) end of the spectrum. The ultraviolet radiation is converted to visible light by a coating of phosphor on the inner surface of the tube. The coating fluoresces: it receives radiant energy at one wavelength (in this case ultraviolet) and emits it with lower energy at another, longer, wavelength (in this case in the form of visible light).

The fluorescent lamp is still the most common form of gas-discharge lighting, although low-pressure sodium lamps are extensively used for street lighting. Other efficient high-power lamps are becoming increasingly widespread. These include the high-pressure sodium lamp (usually pinky or orangey-white in colour) and the high-pressure mercury lamp (bluey-white).

6.2 Pulsating discharge

In a fluorescent lamp, the electrodes are usually connected to the alternating current supply. The voltage across the ends of the tube varies sinusoidally, one electrode carrying alternately a positive and then a negative potential compared to the other. As a result, two discharges within the gas occur with each cycle of the supply. Over most of the length of the tube the light pulsates with a frequency twice that of the supply voltage. In Europe where the electricity supply has a frequency of 50 cycles per second the lamp pulsates 100 times per second (i.e. at 100 Hz). In North America where a 60 Hz supply is used the pulsation has a frequency of 120 Hz. The waveform depends on the constituent phosphors and is often similar to a rectified sine-wave, see Fig. 6.1.

6.3 Luminaires and depth of pulsation

The discharge does not occur evenly along the length of the tube: there are dark spaces in front of the negative electrode (Crooke's and Faraday's dark spaces). At the ends of the tube the light is therefore flickering at the frequency of the electricity supply (typically with 50 or 60 flashes per second) and the flicker is sometimes visible. For this reason fluorescent lamps are often mounted in a box or 'luminaire' with reflective inner surfaces so that light from the ends of the tubes is mixed with light elsewhere within

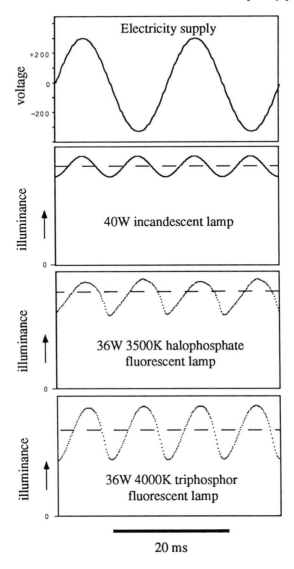

Fig. 6.1 Electricity supply voltage and light output by various electric lamps as a function of time. Light measurements were made using a photodiode with a spectral response resembling that of the eye (i.e. approximating the V_λ curve), and all wavelengths between 400 and 700 nm therefore contributed, with wavelengths near 550 nm contributing most. The photodiode was directed at one end of the halophosphate fluorescent lamp in order to exaggerate the 50 Hz component, and this can be seen as a difference in the size of neighbouring pulsations. (The difference would have been too small to be seen had the light from the entire tube been measured.)

the luminaire, 'diluting' the low-frequency component. The dilution reduces the *modulation depth*, that is, the proportionate amount by which the light varies with time.

Luminaires of this kind are effective at removing most of the modulation at the frequency of the electricity supply, provided the tube is new. Unfortunately, as the tube ages, another source of low-frequency modulation becomes important. One electrode often deteriorates more rapidly than the other, and the discharge when the current is flowing in one direction down the tube may then be less than that when the current flows in the opposite direction. An alternately bright and dim discharge results, providing fluctuation at the frequency of the AC supply. No amount of diffusion within the luminaire will remove it.

Luminaires can also do nothing to remove the pulsation of light that occurs at twice the frequency of the supply. This pulsation varies considerably from one type of lamp to another.

6.4 Varieties of fluorescent lamps

Different fluorescent lamps use different gas mixtures and different phosphor coatings. The extent to which the light output varies at twice the frequency of the supply depends upon these coatings. The pulsation shown in Fig. 6.1 was measured over a range of wavelengths between 400 and 700 nm giving greatest weighting to wavelengths close to 550 nm where the eye is most sensitive. The variation in energy is shown in more detail in Fig. 6.2. Here the energy is shown as a function of wavelength at several instants in time through half of one electricity cycle. The variation is shown for a common lamp with a halophosphate coating of phosphor and also for a more modern lamp that uses different phosphors, similar to those in television – the so-called *triphosphor* lamp. It is obvious that the variation is greater for some wavelengths than for others. For the common lamp (with a halophosphate coating) the pulsation of light is far greater at the short wavelength (blue) end of the visible spectrum. This is because some of the component phosphors exhibit *phosphorescence*, they continue to glow after excitation by the gas discharge, holding some of the light. These phosphors are said to be *persistent*, and the phosphors with long persistence are those that emit light at the long-wavelength end (red) of the spectrum.

The graphs shown in Fig. 6.2 are instantaneous *spectral power distributions*. The graphs can be used to calculate the variation in the energy captured by the photoreceptors of the eye as a function of time. There are four types of photoreceptor: rod receptors (active mainly at twilight levels of illumination) and three types of cone receptors, one sensitive to

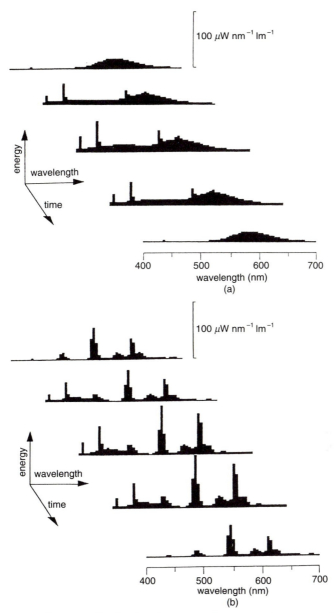

Fig. 6.2 The spectral power distribution from two fluorescent lamps as a function of time. Five distributions are shown at different instants spaced 25 ms apart beginning and ending when the energy from the gas discharge was minimal. (a) White halophosphate lamp; (b) triphosphor lamp. (After Wilkins and Clark 1990.)

Table 6.1 Modulation from fluorescent lamps calculated from spectral power distributions similar to those shown in Fig. 6.1. The lamps are listed by CIE category and correlated colour temperature (CCT). Modulation is calculated as the ratio $(E_{max} - E_{min})/(E_{max} + E_{min}) \times 100\%$ where E_{max} and E_{min} are the maximum and minimum energy, and the engery refers respectively to the luminance (estimated using the V_λ function) and to the energy captured by the photoreceptors and putative neural channels (estimated using the spectral weighting functions due to Hunt 1987[*]). The range of values for both wide and narrow diameter lamps are shown. The narrow diameter lamps have a lower modulation. (After Wilkins and Clark 1990.)

	Halophosphate			Triphosphor	Daylight
	Warm white	White	Cool white		
CIE category	F4	F3	F2	F11	F7
CCT (k)	2900	3500	4000–4200	4000	6500
Luminance	17–20	22	27–31	36–40	>80
L-receptors	14–16	18	23–26	37–42	>80
M-receptors	19–21	24	30–34	34–38	>80
S-receptors	87–94	86	88–95	78–83	>80
L−M channel	15–16	24	48–56	67–84	>80
L+M−2S channel	18–21	22	41–49	54–62	>80

[*]Hunt (1987, 1991) uses the abbreviations, R, G, and B to refer to the L, M, and S receptors, respectively.

long wavelength light (L-receptor), one medium wavelengths (M), and one short (S). The variation in energy captured by these receptors can be calculated from their *spectral sensitivities* (i.e. their sensitivities at different wavelengths), as will now be shown.

6.5 Modulation

The modulation was referred to earlier as the proportionate amount by which the light energy varies with time. It is often expressed as the difference between maximum and minimum energy divided by the sum of the maximum and minimum. This fraction varies from 0 per cent when there is no variation, to 100 per cent when the energy falls to zero each cycle. The variation in the energy captured by the various photoreceptors can be expressed by this fraction, and Table 6.1 lists the percentage modulation characteristics of various types of lamp. It also shows the modulation in *luminance*, which, as we have seen in Chapter 2, is a psychophysically determined function that expresses the brightness sensation. As can be seen, 'warm white' halophosphate lamps give the lowest modulation in luminance, and in the energy captured by the long- and medium-wavelength photoreceptors.

There are anecdotal reports that some people prefer warm white lamps:

In one company strong staff preference for warm white tubes led to the policy of using warm white for all replacements. In practice this often required more tubes to be replaced than were strictly necessary because of the unattractive appearance of mixed tubes in a single fitting ... In a newspaper office refurbished for the introduction of a new editorial computer system lighting levels were higher than intended and half the tubes had to be removed to lower the levels to be more appropriate for VDU use, and again strong staff preference for warm white led to their introduction. However, it was only some of the staff who expressed this view and so the final solution was to allow staff to choose tube type in areas where the strong preference existed. It is usually a minority who express a strong view: others are usually indifferent rather than in favour of cool white. (T. Stewart, Systems Concepts Ltd).

Some of the preferences may reflect the association of warm colours with domestic lighting from incandescent sources (Baron *et al.* 1992). Alternatively they may reflect the influence of the rapid pulsation of light, as will become clear. Despite the preferences, cool white or white lamps are usually installed because they are more efficient, at least in the sense that they give more lumens per watt.

6.6 Physiological consequences of the pulsation in light

6.6.1 Flicker 'fusion'

An intermittent light no longer appears to flicker when the frequency exceeds some limit commonly referred to as a *flicker 'fusion' threshold*. When the light is bright and diffuse and stimulates a large retinal area this threshold can be as high as 90 Hz (i.e. 90 flashes per second). It is rarely higher (Van de Grind *et al.* 1973), although there are exceptional observers who can reliably see flicker at frequencies in excess of 100 Hz. The 'fusion' threshold cannot, however, be taken as a limit above which intermittent light has the same effect as continuous light. First, Berman *et al.* (1991) have recorded the electrical activity of the human retina using electrodes attached to the eye. The electroretinogram showed responses to intermittent light at frequencies higher than 100 Hz. Evidently cells in the human retina resolve high frequencies. Second, Brindley (1962) demonstrated psychophysically that the nervous system resolves intermittent light at frequencies well above the flicker fusion threshold. He stimulated the retina electrically so as to produce the appearance of flashes of light (*phosphenes*). When he increased the frequency of electrical stimulation sufficiently the phosphenes appeared continuous. Brindley combined high-frequency electrical stimulation with stimulation from high-frequency intermittent light. Both the phosphenes and the light stimulation appeared continuous when presented on their own. When the two forms of stimulation were combined and the frequencies were slightly different, however, observers reported seeing the beat between the two. The beat was perceptible when the visual stimulation had a frequency as high as 125 Hz indicating that, at some level, the visual system was resolving light stimulation at this frequency.

6.6.2 Subcortical response to fluorescent lighting

The fluctuations from fluorescent lighting affect subcortical activity in the brain. Eysel and Burandt (1984) recorded from visual neurones in the cat when the animal was looking at a surface subtending 50 deg at the eye, a larger stimulus than is typically used in physiological studies of single neurones. The surface was illuminated by fluorescent light, by incandescent light with the same brightness (time-averaged luminance), or by daylight. Neurones in the *optic tract* (neural pathways from the eyes) and the *lateral geniculate nucleus* of the thalamus (a subcortical visual area) fired twice as strongly under fluorescent illumination than under the incandescent illumination or daylight. Some cells responded to each flash from the fluorescent light, some responded less frequently, but the firing of all cells was *phase-locked* to the light pulsation, that is, the cells all tended to fire just before the light reached its peak. This pattern of activity occurred whether the fluorescent lighting pulsated 100 or 120 times per second. The findings are therefore of importance in countries that use a 50 Hz or 60 Hz electricity supply. It was only when the supply was altered so that the pulsation in the light reached a frequency of 160 Hz that the neurones failed to show phase-locked responding. The luminance of the light did not seem to make much difference over a range of one log unit (a factor of ten). Comparatively little phase-locking was seen in response to incandescent illumination with the same luminance.

Eysel and Burandt did not record from cells in the visual cortex. Cortical cells are thought not to respond to variation in contrast at frequencies in excess of about 20 Hz (Movshon *et al.* 1978). Further, Eysel and Burandt's experiments were performed on cats, they have not been repeated with primates and it is impossible to know whether cells in the human visual system show a similar response to fluorescent light.

Eysel and Burandt pointed out that phase-locked responding similar to that which they recorded in the lateral geniculate nucleus and optic tract should also be seen in other visual structures: those that are connected by short neural chains to the optic tract or lateral geniculate nucleus. Such visual structures include the *superior colliculus*, a body associated with the control of eye movements. It is therefore interesting that high frequency pulsation of light has been shown to interfere with the control of eye movements in human observers.

6.6.3 Eye movements

Wilkins (1986) recorded movements of the eyes across text illuminated by two types of fluorescent light, one conventional, exhibiting the 100 Hz pulsation typical in Europe, and the other with electronic circuitry that produced pulsation at a very high frequency (> 30 kHz), too fast for the retinal neurones. Observers were asked to direct their gaze alternately between two specified letters on the same line in a page of text, and the size of the rapid eye movements (*saccades*) was measured. The saccades were slightly (3–5 per cent) larger under the conventional fluorescent light. The increase in saccade size, though statistically significant, was weak: it accounted for only 4 per cent of the experimental variance.

The effect of pulsating light on eye movements may help to explain the small impairments in visual search observed in a study by Rey and Rey (1963). Over the course of four weeks a complex visual search task was repeatedly performed by five subjects with good vision. Certain letters from a list had to be cancelled if they occurred in a context defined by other neighbouring letters. Before and after periods of 45 min at this task a variety of other measures were taken. These included the simple reaction time to a visual stimulus, and the frequency at which a series of brief flashes appeared continuous (flicker fusion). Under conventional fluorescent lighting (50 Hz circuitry), performance of the visual search task was slightly poorer than under fluorescent lighting with very high frequency circuitry. The difference between measures taken before and after the task was greater under the conventional lighting.

Rey and Rey reviewed a number of early studies of the effects of fluorescent lighting on vision and visual perception. The effects of the pulsations were sometimes inconsistent but were generally detrimental. The effects were uniformly small.

If fluorescent lighting had major effects on visual perception or the control of eye-movements these would have been noticed and would have given rise to complaints. Complaints there certainly have been, but concerning headaches and eye-strain rather than any visual or perceptual phenomena.

6.7 Links with headaches and eye-strain

At the anecdotal level there is much to suggest that fluorescent lighting induces headaches in a few people, particularly those with migraine. Some people are severely affected and have to avoid fluorescent lighting as much as possible. Pulsating light may be one possible cause for these complaints as will now be shown.

6.7.1 Electrophysiological evidence

When an observer looks at a flickering light, the electrical brain activity (electroencephalograph) over the *occiput* at the back of the head shows a response at the same frequency as the light. Sometimes this response is so large as to be visible against the other brain rhythms in the electroencephalograph tracing, but it is usually necessary to average the electrical response to many flashes before it can be measured. This *evoked potential* results from the electrical field generated when large populations of neurones fire in synchrony, see Section 4.3. Golla and Winter (1959) showed that in persons suffering episodic headaches, but not in controls, the amplitude of the response to intermittent light was greater at flash frequencies of 20 Hz than at lower frequencies, and they termed this the *H-response*, see Section 3.6.

Their findings have since been replicated, notably by Lehtonen (1974), Jonkman and Lelieveld (1981), and Nyrke and Lang (1982), see Winter (1987) for review. Brundrett (1974) investigated the response at high flash frequencies. He measured the decrease in the amplitude of the evoked potential as the frequency of the flickering light increased. In a small sample of headache sufferers he showed that the decrease with frequency was less than in controls, suggesting that the headache sufferers were in some way unusually sensitive to high-frequency flicker.

6.7.2 A survey of office workers

A field study by Wilkins *et al.* (1989) has now shown that the pulsating light from conventional fluorescent lighting is indeed responsible for headaches and eye-strain: in fact the study suggests that more than half the headaches suffered by office workers may be attributable to the lighting.

Staff in a government legal department were asked to keep diaries in which they recorded the occurrence of headache and eye-strain week by week over a period of more than six months. The offices were lit by halophosphate fluorescent lamps (mainly cool white) incorporating one of two types of circuit. The first was conventional choke circuitry and resulted in the usual pulsation in light. The second type was high-frequency (32 kHz) electronic circuitry that greatly reduced the 100-per-second pulsations. Because the lighting differed only with respect to the circuitry hidden in the casing it was possible to undertake a *double-blind* study: a study in which all participants, including those collecting the data, were unaware which type of fluorescent lighting they were exposed to. A double-blind procedure is important in any study of this kind where responses can be influenced by what people believe as much as by what is actually the case.

The government department in which the study took place had a large number of small offices receiving little daylight. The staff undertook close visual work almost entirely without the use of computer displays.

The conventional and the new lighting differed in the speed with which the lamps ignited: the new lighting ignited instantaneously whereas the conventional lighting lit only after a few preliminary flashes. A third type of fitting was therefore introduced. This incorporated electronic ignition so that the tube ignited rapidly, but in all other respects the light was conventional: it pulsated in the usual way. The staff exposed to conventional lighting with rapid ignition constituted a control group who experienced a visible change in the lighting installation but no change in the 100-per-second fluctuations. By comparing this group with the other two it was therefore possible to know whether the reporting of headaches or eye-strain was affected by the speed of lamp ignition, or indeed the noticeable change in installation.

The three types of fluorescent lighting were allocated at random and were changed over halfway through the winter period during which the data were collected.

There was no difference in the incidence of headaches or eye-strain under the two forms of conventional lighting, suggesting that the speed of ignition had no discernible effect on symptoms. Under the new type of lighting, however, the incidence of headaches and eye-strain was more than halved. People who reported frequent headaches tended to report frequent eye-strain as well. The correlation between the two types of pain is shown in Fig. 6.3. Although the correlation is significant, it is not large, and for this reason eye-strain was analysed separately from headaches.

The change in the incidence of headaches and eye-strain as a function of lighting was statistically significant, but the result was based on only a few participants. Fortunately the sample size could be increased by considering the relatively large number of participants whose lighting remained unaltered (it would have cost too much to alter all the lamps in the building). These people experienced conventional lighting throughout the period of the study and they provided a baseline control. By including these individuals the size of the sample of people experiencing conventional fluorescent lighting before and after the changeover was increased to 91. The distribution of the incidence of eye-strain in this group is shown in Fig. 6.4. The distribution is highly skewed: a few people suffered considerably, most did not suffer at all.

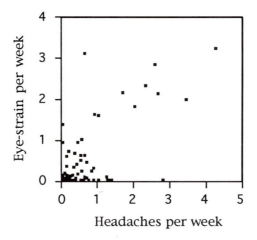

Fig. 6.3 Scattergram showing the correlation between reports of eye-strain and headache in a survey of office workers. (After Wilkins *et al.* 1989.)

This figure also shows for comparison the corresponding distributions for the group who experienced the new high-frequency lighting. Notice that the 'tails' of the distributions are shorter: there were fewer people who suffered often. The distributions for the second half of the study (after the lighting was changed over) were very similar to those in Fig. 6.4. The corresponding distributions for headaches were similar to those for eye-strain.

The building was six storeys high and although the offices all had windows they overlooked buildings of similar height. The amount of daylight entering the window therefore increased with the height of the office above the ground. On a sunny day the increase averaged about 80 lux per storey, measured at the occupant's desk. The incidence of headaches amongst those exposed to conventional fluorescent lighting decreased with the height of the office above the ground. The height of the office was not correlated with occupation or any other factor likely to have influenced the reporting of eye-strain or headache. Eye-strain and headaches may therefore have been affected by the availability of natural light. Even when the fluorescent lighting was turned on, daylight would have 'diluted' the fluctuations in illumination.

Evidently the imperceptible fluctuations in conventional fluorescent lighting can provoke eye-strain and headaches.

Timers were inserted in a random sample of the light fittings to measure the total time for which the lights were turned on. On average the new fluorescent lighting was turned on for 30 per cent longer than the conventional lighting, suggesting that people preferred it.

As mentioned above, conventional fluorescent lighting fluctuates mainly

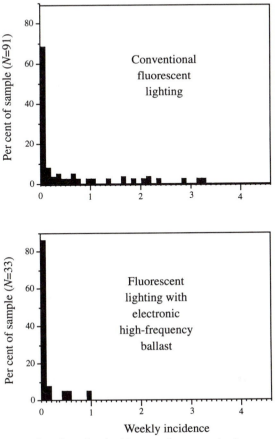

Fig. 6.4 Histograms showing the incidence of eye-strain in a survey of office workers. The survey compared the weekly incidence of these complaints when the offices were lit by conventional fluorescent fittings and by outwardly identical fittings incorporating circuitry that removed most of the 100 Hz and 50 Hz pulsations (high-frequency ballast). The histograms show the incidence of eye-strain for the first half of the study (before the lighting was changed over). The corresponding histograms for eye-strain after the change and for headaches before and after the change were very similar, although different subjects contributed. (After Wilkins *et al.* 1989.)

at a frequency twice that of the AC supply, but also slightly at the same frequency as the supply. In the above study, the lamps were all encased in luminaires which reduced the 50 Hz component to a few per cent. Although it remains possible that the 50 Hz component was responsible for the headaches, it seems unlikely.

Neither the 100-per-second nor the 50-per-second fluctuation is usually visible, which suggests that pulsating illumination is capable of inducing headache even when people are unaware of the fluctuations. None of the study participants blamed the lighting for their headaches.

6.8 Links with agoraphobia

Some people have an irrational fear of going out (*agoraphobia*) and tend to stay at home. They often suffer attacks of sudden and extreme fear which they are unable to control (*panic attacks*). During the course of clinical work I noted that a substantial proportion of these patients reported that fluorescent lighting precipitated their attacks. Watts and Wilkins (1989) therefore undertook three questionnaire studies asking volunteers to report the stimuli, visual and otherwise, that precipitated their panic. The responses to these questionnaires confirmed the original clinical impression. Certain specific visual stimuli tended to be reported as precipitating panic. The visual stimuli responsible were those that provoke visual discomfort. The association with panic was confined to these visual stimuli and was seen only in patients with agoraphobia and not in normal controls or patients with other types of phobia.

Following this study, Hazell and Wilkins (1990) tested agoraphobic volunteers in their own homes under three types of lighting: conventional fluorescent, high-frequency fluorescent, and incandescent. Patients reported more symptoms of panic under the fluorescent lighting than under the incandescent, but the responses to the two types of fluorescent lighting were similar. The patients were unaware that two types of fluorescent lighting were under comparison, and the examiner was unaware as to which type of fluorescent lighting was which. She took the patient's pulse as part of the examination, and the pulse rate was higher under the conventional fluorescent lighting, see Fig. 6.5. The heart rate did not differ under the two relatively steady forms of lighting (incandescent and high-frequency fluorescent).

The author has since seen several patients who have developed an aversion to fluorescent lighting following a period of intense work at a visual display terminal. This aversion has led to a tendency to stay at home. Most shops and offices are lit by gas-discharge lighting of one kind or another, and it is difficult to leave one's home without exposing oneself to pulsating light, even during the day. Perhaps certain visually sensitive people can develop agoraphobia partly for this reason, although it seems most unlikely that fluorescent lighting is a major direct cause of agoraphobia. Instead the anxiety may increase awareness of minor bodily symptoms, such as those

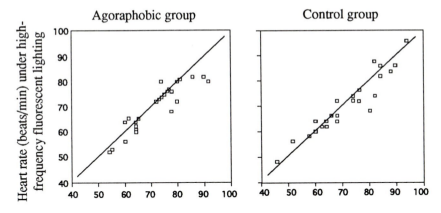

Heart rate (beats min⁻¹) under conventional fluorescent lighting

Fig. 6.5 Heart rate of female volunteers with agoraphobia and controls examined under conventional fluorescent lighting and fluorescent lighting controlled by circuitry that reduces the fluctuations in light intensity. Each point represents a person, its position determined by her heart rate under the two forms of lighting. Note that the points tend to lie below the diagonal indicating an increased heart rate under conventional fluorescent light. (After Hazell and Wilkins 1990.)

induced by fluorescent lighting, and these symptoms may then be elaborated cognitively.

6.9 Physiological mechanisms for discomfort

The data considered thus far suggest that the high frequency pulsations from electric lighting are resolved by the visual system and cause headache, eye-strain, and perhaps also symptoms prodromal to panic. In Chapter 4 it was shown that the visual stimuli that provoke seizures in patients with photosensitive epilepsy are those that, in others, provoke feelings of discomfort. It was inferred that the visual stimuli responsible for discomfort are those that give rise to an intense physiological activation of visual neurones. The activation may perhaps be increased by stimuli that compromise the normal computational processes underlying vision, such as those involved in the control of eye movements. Any visual stimulus that increases the number of eye movements necessary for a visual task might be expected to increase the neuronal work involved in seeing. Kennedy and Murray (1991) have demonstrated that when text is illuminated by light pulsating

100 times per second, the number of eye movements necessary for reading can be as much as doubled. Perhaps the discomfort associated with the use of fluorescent lighting can be attributed to the effects of the pulsation on the control of eye movements.

Curiously, complaints about fluorescent lighting are not often made by people with photosensitive epilepsy. These people seem to complain of lighting much less frequently than those with migraine, for example. Moreover, fluorescent lighting does not appear to induce EEG abnormalities in photosensitive patients. Binnie *et al.* (1979b) caused a fluorescent lamp to malfunction and produce far more fluctuation at 50 and 100 Hz than is usual. They recorded the EEG of patients with photosensitive epilepsy during exposure to this flicker but failed to observe any epileptiform activity. Of course, they recorded the EEG for short periods only, and it remains possible that long-term exposure might increase the incidence of epileptiform abnormalities, an increase which would be measurable only by long-term recordings. On the other hand, it is also possible that the apparent differences in the susceptibility of persons with migraine and epilepsy are due to a basic difference in mechanism. In Chapter 4 it was argued that strong physiological activation was necessary for seizures and headaches, but in Chapter 2 it was shown that seizures occurred only when the resulting excitation was synchronized (Section 2.3.5). This hypothesis would predict a difference in the susceptibility to fluorescent lighting amongst persons with migraine and those with epilepsy, as will now be shown.

It will be recalled that Eysel and Burandt's (1984) recordings from the optic tract and lateral geniculate nucleus showed that under fluorescent light, cells were responding at about twice the rate at which they would in response to steady light, and that their firing was phase-locked to each pulse of light. In other words, the excitation in subcortical systems was increased, and it was synchronized. As has already been noted, cortical neurones are thought to be unable to resolve stimulation at high temporal frequencies. Fluorescent lighting is therefore unlikely to affect synchronization at a cortical level. It might nevertheless increase the overall level of cortical excitation as a non-specific consequence of the unnatural subcortical activity interfering with the control of eye movements.

If seizures start in the visual cortex in response to massive synchronized excitation, as hypothesized in Chapter 2, then they are not likely to be triggered by fluorescent lighting. On the other hand, fluorescent lighting or any other visual stimulation that increases the overall level of excitation (without any particular synchronization) should increase the probability of headaches and eye-strain. The differences between the visual stimulation responsible for seizures and that responsible for other adverse effects such as headaches may therefore be attributed to the part played by the synchronization of cortical activity in the induction of seizures.

6.10 Remedial measures

Several steps can be taken to minimize the pulsation of light, and to reduce the effects of any pulsation that remains. Ideally, of course, the circuitry controlling the lighting should be changed to a type that does not generate a significant modulation at 100 Hz. High-frequency electronic ballast consumes 40 per cent less power and emits only 5 per cent less light, but it is twice as expensive as the conventional circuitry. The people who build offices are not usually those who run them, and so the cheaper running costs from the new circuitry do not necessarily provide the incentive for change. A change to high-frequency circuitry is expensive and is usually only considered when a major lighting refit is justified by other considerations.

Incandescent uplighters can provide an alternative to fluorescent lighting. Uplighters stand on the floor or hang from a wall and shine their light on the ceiling. They are useful for individual sufferers because they do not necessitate changing the office lighting installation: the units simply plug into wall outlets. Some uplighters use high-pressure gas discharge lamps, but those that are sold for the domestic market have high-power 240 V tungsten halogen lamps. The resulting illumination is diffuse and bright enough to substitute for fluorscent lamps. Although the light is yellow it has a greater contribution from short wavelengths than is available from more conventional incandescent sources. The light does not flicker, even when dimmed, because the thick filament retains the heat from one half-cycle of the electricity supply to the next. A few of the small unshielded tungsten–halogen lamps may emit sufficient ultraviolet energy to be deemed a health hazard (McKinlay *et al.* 1989), but the main disadvantages of the uplighters are that the lamps are less efficient than gas-discharge lamps, and produce far more heat. They are not in general a cost-effective solution.

The pulsation from fluorescent lighting depends on the type of lamp. Narrow warm-white halophosphate lamps show the lowest peak – peak modulation (17–18 per cent). Triphosphor lamps show a modulation twice as great (see Table 6.1). It may be worth considering refitting warm-white lamps in installations that have triphosphor lamps.

If the above solutions are not practical, it is important for headache sufferers to work near a window. If no daylight is available then relief can sometimes be obtained from tinted spectacle lenses.

6.10.1 Tinted lenses for fluorescent lighting?

As can be seen from Fig. 6.2, the pulsation from a typical (halophosphate) lamp is greatest at the short-wavelength (blue) end of the visible spectrum: the red light remains relatively steady. Spectacles with tinted lenses that selectively absorb short wavelength light therefore reduce the pulsation.

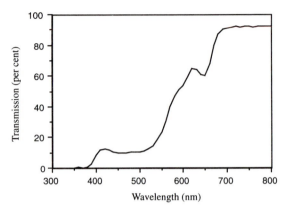

Fig. 6.6 The transmission characteristics of spectacles that remove about 30 per cent of the pulsations from conventional 'white' and 'cool white' fluorescent lamps, whilst avoiding any pronounced distortion of colour. (After Wilkins and Wilkinson 1991.)

The greatest reduction in pulsation would be achieved by a filter that passed no light with a wavelength less than 600 nm. Such a filter would not transmit much light and would be very red, and interfere with colour perception. Some compromise between the competing demands for adequate colour perception and reduction in pulsation has to be achieved. A new ophthalmic tint (*Comfort 41®*) has been designed by Wilkins and Wilkinson (1991) and provides one possible compromise.[1] It has a rose – brown appearance.[2] Figure 6.6 shows the transmission of the tint as a function of wavelength. Figure 6.7 shows the effect of the tint in reducing the pulsation of light from various types of fluorescent lighting. As can be seen, with a 'white' halophosphate lamp it transmits about one third of the light and it reduces pulsation by about one third. It also reduces the modulation in the opponent colour channels. Notice that the effects with halophosphate lamps differ from those with triphosphor lamps. Because triphosphor lamps show a greater modulation at both short and long wavelengths, a filter that transmits mainly long-wavelength light can act to enhance the modulation reaching the eye, rather than reduce it. The notch in the transmission curve at around 650 nm is an attempt to reduce this effect as much as possible.

---

[1] It is marketed by Cambridge Optical Group Ltd, Bar Hill, Cambridge.
[2] The first mention of 'rose-coloured spectacles' was metaphorical. Hughes (1861) in *Tom Brown at Oxford* (II, 102): 'Oxford was a sort of Utopia to Captain . . . to behold towers and quadrangles, and chapels—through rose-coloured spectacles.' The French say 'voir tout en rose', prefering metaphorical spectacles.

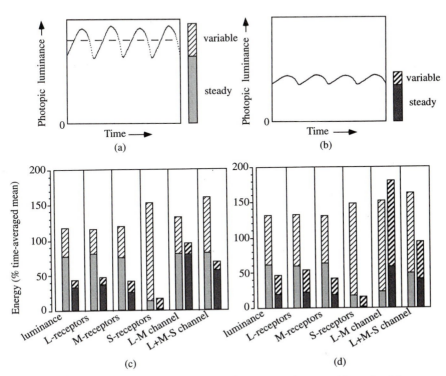

Fig. 6.7 The pulsation of light from two fluorescent lamps with and without an ophthalmic tint having the transmission shown in Fig. 6.6. (a) The modulation in light energy from a white halophosphate fluorescent lamp is expressed as a steady component to which a variable component (shown by hatching) is added. The time-averaged output is shown by the broken line. When the ophthalmic tint is worn and the patient looks at a white surface, the steady and variable components (shown by the vertical bar chart) are both reduced, as in (b), but the relative proportions of steady and variable light energy are also changed. In (c) the steady and variable components are shown by solid and hatched bars respectively, both without and with the ophthalmic tint (left and right vertical bars respectively). The photopic luminance is shown in the first pair of bar graphs. The tint results in a 30 per cent reduction in modulation. The equivalent graphs for the light energy captured by the long-, medium-, and short-wavelength receptors are shown next. The last two graphs show data for the putative colour-opponent channels of Hunt (1987). In (d) the corresponding graphs for a triphosphor lamp are shown. (After Wilkins and Wilkinson 1991.)

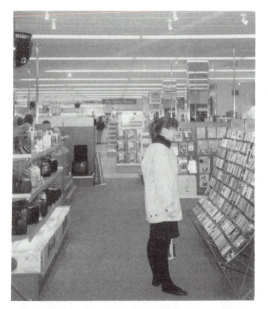
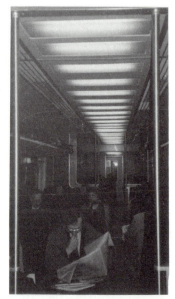
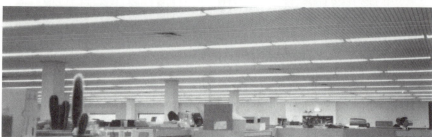

Fig. 6.8 Examples of typical lighting installations, showing the spatially periodic pattern of light and dark contours.

The clinical effects of the tint were investigated in a small-scale but placebo-controlled study by Good *et al.* (1991). Children with migraine were given either the rose tint or an alternative blue tint that transmitted a similar amount of light (i.e. had similar *photopic transmission*). The tints were allocated randomly. The children reported that both tints reduced photophobia during attacks, but only the rose one decreased the number of attacks. In unpublished open trials, the lens was reported to reduce headaches in office workers who used visual display units (Wilkinson, personal communication). One possible mechanism for such a reduction has emerged in recent unpublished EEG studies of photosensitive epilepsy.

A patient with photosensitive epilepsy had reported seizures when working at a visual display unit. When examined in the EEG laboratory, there was no epileptiform activity unless he used the display under fluorescent lighting. The display was a VGA monitor which had a refresh rate of 70 Hz, and therefore produced a low-frequency beat with the lighting. Flicker at low frequencies is known to induce epileptiform activity, see Chapter 2. The *Comfort 41®* lens prevented EEG discharges when the visual display unit was used (Wilkins and Kasteleijn, personal observations).

6.11 Spatial layout of lighting

Thus far in this chapter we have considered only the temporal aspects of electric lighting, and the manner in which the rapid pulsation of light can be a source of discomfort, and even of seizures. In previous chapters we have seen how the spatial properties of visual stimuli can cause discomfort. We now turn briefly to the spatial properties of lighting. Figure 6.8 shows examples of typical lighting installations and it illustrates the way in which rows of luminaires can produce patterns of stripes. The luminaires are usually positioned in this way in order to make the distribution of light as even as possible and to rationalize the trunking carrying the electrical cables. If the luminaires emit light to the side and a low ceiling is viewed obliquely, the spatial frequency can be in the adverse range, see Fig. 6.8. These effects are reduced if the luminaires are flush with the ceiling and baffles direct their light downward. Unfortunately the baffles themselves often form stripes. In the next chapter we will discuss the rapid pulsation of light from other sources, televisions and computer displays, and show how the pulsation is combined with other types of pattern.

7 Electronic displays

Electronic displays usually use a cathode ray tube. The image pulsates in brightness, the top of the display being lit before the bottom. The flicker may not be noticeable, but it can induce seizures. The seizures may be prevented by viewing with one eye using selective polarized occlusion. When text is displayed, the pulsation interferes with saccadic suppression and increases the number of rapid eye movements required for reading. This may be one reason for the complaints of eye-strain and headache associated with the use of computer displays.

In the following chapter we will briefly describe some of the techniques involved in the presentation of visual information by electronic means. We will examine the impact of the technology on visual discomfort and discuss the physiological mechanisms involved.

Electronic displays are now found in every walk of life. They are responsible for most of the information exchange between humans and machines. The range of technology used in such displays is very large. Some use liquid crystals that change their reflectance in response to an electric field, others use gas plasma that emits light in much the same way as the fluorescent lamp. However, one form of technology predominates over all others: the cathode ray tube. The tube is of glass, usually conical in shape, with electrodes at the point of the cone and a phosphor screen at the opposite end. Electrons are 'boiled off' a heated electrode, and are focused and accelerated by a strong electric or magnetic field towards the screen. The screen has a coating on the inner surface of the glass, containing a photochemical that fluoresces when struck by the beam of electrons. Electrons in this phosphor coating are 'knocked' from one orbit to another with a lower energy, emitting photons, and creating a spot of light. The beam of electrons is deflected with a rapidly varying electric or magnetic field so that it repeatedly zigzags down the screen in a pattern of horizontal lines, known as a *raster*. As it does so the intensity of the beam is altered so that the spot of light 'paints' the image. When the entire screen has been scanned, the beam flies back to the top and repeats the raster scan.

7.1 Television

Most televisions use a cathode ray tube (CRT). The time the beam takes to scan from the top to the bottom of the screen depends on the television standard: in Europe it takes about 1/50th second and in North America about 1/60th.

Odd-numbered lines are drawn on one scan and even-numbered lines on the next, so that two interlacing series of lines are drawn alternately. Each line therefore appears once every two scans. If the scans are repeated 50 times a second, as in Europe, each line is drawn only 25 times per second. The scan therefore gives rise to a pattern similar to stripes that alternate between black and white at 25 Hz. As we shall see later, it is this aspect of a television picture more than any other that has been responsible for the induction of epileptic seizures.

In a colour television the picture is scanned as described above, but instead of one electron gun there are three. The three beams are interrupted by a *shadow mask* close to the screen. The mask has small holes so as to create tiny points of light, some red, some green, and some blue, due to three different coatings of phosphor. As the screen is scanned the position of the points follows the zigzag of the raster. The intensity of each colour varies so as to create a coloured picture.

7.2 Television epilepsy

A large proportion of patients with photosensitive epilepsy suffer their first seizure when watching television, often when they are close to the screen. Many patients suffer seizures *only* under these circumstances.

When television-induced seizures were first described they were attributed to malfunction of the television. Such malfunction was common in the early days, when the picture would frequently become unstable and 'roll', introducing a low-frequency flicker. As the number of reports increased it became apparent that seizures could also be induced by a set that was functioning quite normally.

Stefansson *et al.* (1977) noted that patients with television epilepsy tended also to be pattern-sensitive. Eventually it became clear that the reason for the association with pattern sensitivity was the pattern created by the raster scan. Wilkins *et al.* (1979*b*) recorded the EEG while patients watched one of three televisions:

(1) a television with a small (0.27 m) screen;

(2) a television with a large screen (roughly twice the size); and

(3) the large screen covered with a cardboard mask bearing a central aperture the same size as the small screen, see Fig. 7.1.

The small screen and the masked screen had the same size: half that of the large screen. The size of the lines on the large screen was the same as that

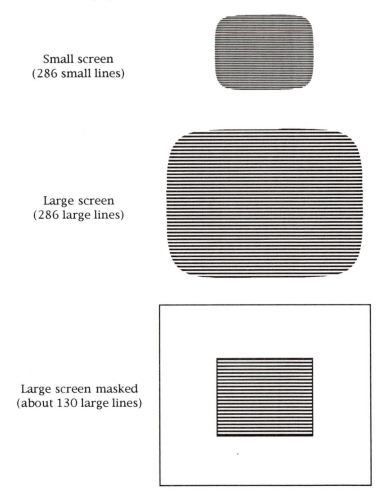

Small screen
(286 small lines)

Large screen
(286 large lines)

Large screen masked
(about 130 large lines)

Fig. 7.1 Screens used to assess separately the effects of line subtense and screen subtense.

on the masked screen and twice that on the small. In this way the effects of screen size and line size could be estimated separately. Viewing distance was progressively reduced, increasing the retinal size of the image of the television until epileptiform EEG activity appeared. The television was then immediately turned off, to avoid a seizure.

For the majority of patients, epileptiform EEG activity appeared at distances that were the same for the large screen and the masked screen, suggesting that the retinal size of the component lines was the critical feature. The activity appeared only when the patient was close to the screen, suggesting that the retinal image of the component lines had to be greater than a certain size, that is, their spatial frequency had to be low enough.

When the patients were examined using the conventional photostimulator (a xenon 'strobe' light used for EEG examinations), epileptiform EEG activity appeared only at flash frequencies lower than 50 Hz, confirming that the 25 Hz line interlace was the feature responsible for the epileptiform activity. Patterns of stripes that vibrate or repeatedly reverse their phase are most likely to evoke epileptiform EEG abnormalities at frequencies close to 20 Hz, see Section 2.2.2.

Although the 25 Hz interlace was the mechanism responsible for epileptiform activity in the majority of cases, there were a few patients for whom this explanation was insufficient. These were the patients who were sensitive at normal viewing distances. At these distances the component lines on the screen were difficult to see, and the spatial frequency of the lines was too high for any epileptiform response from the pattern. For these patients the large screen gave rise to epileptiform activity at a viewing distance twice that for the other two screens, suggesting that the retinal size of the screen rather than the component lines was the relevant factor. These results are exactly what would be expected if, for these patients, it was the 50 Hz flicker from the scan that was responsible for the epileptiform activity, and not the 25 Hz flicker from the lines. When examined with diffuse intermittent light from the photostimulator the patients did indeed exhibit sensitivity at frequencies as high as 50 Hz.

The findings of the study are therefore quite clear. A few photosensitive patients are sensitive to flicker at high frequencies and are sensitive to television at normal viewing distances because of the 50 Hz screen refresh rate. The majority are sensitive to flicker only at lower frequencies and are at risk from television only when they are close to the screen, when the 25 Hz line interlace pattern has a sufficiently low *spatial* frequency.

There is some suggestion that the prevalence of television epilepsy is lower in North America where the television standard uses a 60 Hz screen refresh rate and a 30 Hz line refresh rate (Jeavons and Harding 1975).

7.3 Implications for treatment

The implications for treatment are obvious. Patients with photosensitive epilepsy who are pattern-sensitive, but who are not sensitive to 50 Hz flicker should be able to watch television from a normal viewing distance. They should avoid getting closer than a distance three times the width of the screen. If they have to get close to the set they should cover one eye with the palm of a hand so as to prevent any intermittent light reaching the retina of that eye. Monocular stimulation is much less likely to cause seizures, see Chapter 2.

Televisions with a diametric measurement smaller than 0.3 m are less of a risk than those with a large screen. Even at close viewing distances the lines cannot be seen clearly enough to have a harmful effect.

Patients who are sensitive to 50 Hz flicker are at risk of a seizure at normal viewing distances. These patients may benefit from some form of monocular occlusion that prevents all the flicker reaching one eye. An eye patch is cheap but usually unacceptable. A more selective and cosmetic occlusion can be achieved in the following way. A sheet of polarizer can be placed over the television screen, so that any light from the television is polarized with a vertical axis of polarization. The patient can wear glasses with one lens polarized vertically and the other horizontally. The glasses look like normal Polaroid® sunglasses but have the effect of preventing the light from the television from reaching one eye. Everything apart from the television can be seen normally, but the television screen appears normal to one eye and black to the other. This form of treatment can prevent seizures quite effectively (Wilkins and Lindsay 1985). Circular polarizers are available which maintain the occlusion regardless of head position. Unfortunately, they are expensive and it has not proved possible to develop this treatment commercially.

Televisions with a liquid crystal display are becoming available. Some use a so-called '*active matrix*' screen, that holds the picture from one scan to the next, and minimizes the flicker. In principle, these televisions should present no risk for patients with epilepsy, and recent EEG studies have shown that patients who are sensitive to conventional television can watch these televisions with no risk (Kasteleijn, personal communication). Televisions with high-frequency refresh rates (100 Hz) are also now available. Again, these should present less of a hazard to patients with epilepsy. Unfortunately, it is still common practice to use flashing graphics as part of the programme material, particularly in cartoons, and sometimes the flashing is in the epileptogenic range.

7.4 Television headaches

Some people, often those with migraine, find that television viewing can make their eyes feel tired and bring on a headache. Sometimes these symptoms can be relieved by the simple expedient of covering the screen with a sheet of dark plastic (about 50 per cent transmission) or with nylon mesh sold for use with computer display terminals. This reduces the brightness of the screen without making the picture more difficult to see, in fact the visibility of the picture may actually be enhanced. This is because light from the surroundings which normally 'dilutes' the television picture has to pass through the filter twice, once before reflection from the surface of the phosphor, and once afterwards. Light from the television picture passes through the filter only once. The contrast of the picture is therefore enhanced but its brightness reduced. Anecdotally, the adverse effects of flicker seem to depend on brightness, and can be reduced by reducing the brightness of the television picture in this way. Unfortunately, no formal studies have explored these issues.

7.5 Computer displays

As already described, computer displays usually use a cathode ray tube. The screen is usually (though not always) scanned in a raster of horizontal lines. The lines differ from those on television in that they are seldom interlaced: all lines, both odd and even, are usually drawn on all scans. Furthermore, the rate at which the screen is refreshed is usually greater than that for television (the difference in the scan frequency is one reason why visual display terminals appear to flicker when viewed on television). The higher refresh rate and the absence of line-interlace mean that seizures from computer displays are rare, although they *do* occur. There is the possibility, discussed in Section 6.10, that the pulsating light from a computer display may interact with that from gas-discharge lighting and induce seizures. Although seizures from computer displays do occur, they are rare, particularly compared with the complaints of visual discomfort which are commonplace. Some possible reasons will now be described.

7.6 Saccadic suppression

Cathode ray tube displays are usually scanned at frequencies between 50 and 100 Hz. When the eyes make a rapid jerk (saccade) they move so quickly that there is time for only one or perhaps two scans of the screen during the eye movement. Briefly presented visual stimuli of this kind can be seen despite the motion of the eye. This was demonstrated in an experiment by Matin *et al.* (1972) who flashed a vertical slit of light during the course of a 4-degree saccade and found that, when the flash was short, observers reported an elongated smear to one side of the slit. As flash duration increased, the perceived length of the smear increased, reaching a maximum at 20 ms. As flash duration increased further, the length of the smear decreased, and it disappeared when the flash duration was similar to that of the eye movement. In other words, for longer flash durations the 'in-flight' retinal stimulation was not perceived. It was as if the image appearing after the eye movement masked the image during the eye movement. It is this *saccadic suppression* that is responsible for the fact that we are normally unaware of the visual image that sweeps across the retina every time our eyes make a saccade. The mechanisms of suppression involve masking, and they break down when the visual scene is intermittently illuminated, as in a cathode ray tube display. Contours from the display can therefore appear momentarily at anomalous locations in space each time an eye movement is made (Neary and Wilkins 1989).

As mentioned above, computer displays are usually scanned by a raster, a series of horizontal sweeps across the screen. The sweeps start at the top of the screen and progress to the bottom. Material displayed at the top of the screen, being lit earlier, can appear momentarily to the left of material from the bottom of the screen when the eyes make a saccade from left to right. When the eyes move in the opposite direction, material at the top appears to the right. There can be a momentary bending or 'shearing' of vertical contours in the direction of the eye movement. The bending can readily be seen if a thick vertical line is created on the surface of a cathode ray tube display (one with a short-persistence phosphor). When the observer makes a saccade across the line, a ghost-like image appears momentarily, leaning in the direction of the eye movement. The distortion is less noticeable when vertical contours are accompanied by other contours that create a 'good figure'. For example, a vertical line tends not to appear to shear when accompanied by a horizontal and oblique line that together create a triangle. The 'goodness of figure' provides for a more stable percept, but one that can still appear to jump with each eye movement (Neary and Wilkins 1989). A column of numbers, or a vertical menu are examples of more realistic configurations: they have vertical edges that can be unstable as a result of the 'shear' from intra-saccadic images. The fleeting intra-saccadic percepts that result may be merely annoying, or they may have a more destructive role, interfering with the control of eye movements.

7.7 Corrective saccades

When the eyes make a large saccade, the movement is usually followed by one or more small corrective saccades that can serve to bring the point of regard closer to the desired position. The momentary instability in the visual world that can accompany each large saccade may affect both the saccade itself and the subsequent saccades. In two studies by Wilkins (1986), observers were asked to change their point of regard repeatedly, looking first at one specified letter in a page of text, and then at another letter on the same line. When the text was displayed on a screen with a 50

Hz scan the saccades were larger than when the screen was refreshed 100 times per second. There were also more corrective movements on the 50 Hz screen. A subsequent study by Kennedy and Murray (1991) used a more natural reading task. They required subjects to read a sentence followed by a word, and to decide whether the word was present in the sentence. They measured the number of saccades made during the task when the screen was lit continuously, and when it was lit repeatedly 50 or 100 times per second. The intermittently illuminated screens were associated with a greater number of eye movements. For some subjects the number of eye movements was more than doubled.

7.8 Modulation depth

Annoying perceptual effects and disturbance of eye movements depend not only on the nature of the spatial configuration displayed and the frequency with which the screen is refreshed, but also on the modulation depth of the pulsating light. The screen emits light because its coating of phosphor is excited by the electron beam. The excitation is very brief but the phosphor continues to emit light for some time after excitation. This *persistence* varies from phosphor to phosphor. Some short-persistence phosphors lose most of their light within microseconds, whereas other so-called 'long-persistence' phosphors lose only about half their light in 16 milliseconds, the duration of one refresh cycle on a typical 60 Hz display. The persistence or after-glow of the phosphor affects the modulation of light from the screen, and this in turn affects the visibility of intra-saccadic stimulation.

Figure 7.2 shows the time-course of illumination from two commonly used phosphors, both green. The screens appear equally bright when the maximum luminance of the long-persistence phosphor is very much less than that of the short. Even when the peak luminances are equated and the colour appearances matched by means of a green filter, the momentary bending of vertical contours is seen only on screens with the short-persistence phosphor. This is presumably because stimulation during a saccade is visible only when it is brief (Matin *et al.* 1972). Neary and Wilkins (1989) measured eye movements across displays with short- or long-persistence phosphors and with a 60 Hz refresh rate. There were more corrective saccades when the screen phosphor had short-persistence than when the persistence was long.

7.9 Visibility of flicker

Occasionally when several screens are visible in close proximity, those in peripheral vision will appear to flicker (this is often noticeable in TV rental

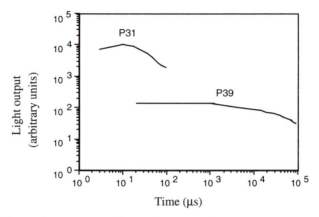

Fig. 7.2 The decay characteristics of two phosphors. A photomultiplier collected the light from a single pixel on the screen of a monitor with a P31 (short-persistence) phosphor and the screen of a similar monitor with a P39 (long-persistence) phosphor. Note the logarithmic coordinates. (After Neary and Wilkins (1989). Courtesy of IBM UK Ltd.)

shops), but generally the scan frequencies are too high for flicker to be perceptible. This may be partly because we have adapted to the top-down direction of the scan. Corbett and White (1976) reported that the flicker from a television display was more perceptible if the display was scanned from bottom to top, rather than in the conventional downwards direction. Thompson (1985) extended their observations, showing that this increase in the perceptibility of flicker depended upon the number of hours of television viewing in previous weeks.

7.10 Precision of eye movement in relation to task performance

We can absorb the information from a picture with a series of saccadic eye movements directed at points of interest, but the exact positioning of the eyes is usually of less importance than in reading, when a series of accurately positioned eye movements is required. One of the important differences between computer displays and television is that the former usually display text, and the disruption of saccadic control by light pulsation can have a greater effect. As mentioned earlier, Kennedy and Murray (1991) presented a sentence followed by a single word and required subjects to report whether the word appeared in the sentence. The intermittent illumination (even at frequencies as high as 100 Hz) gave rise to a twofold increase in saccades amongst those who read with careful attention to the orthographic features of the text (skilled typists). The increase was less marked amongst students who read rapidly for gist. This might be one reason why reading is slower and more proof-reading errors are missed on VDUs as compared with paper (Wilkinson and Robinshaw 1987).

Text is a potentially confusing spatial arrangement of characters with highly similar contours. The eyes move through this maze under the control of a system which uses only the global properties of the image, as we saw in Chapter 5, but precise positioning of the eyes may be necessary for optimal reading (Kennedy and Murray 1991). If words are closely spaced, the global information may be ambiguous, which may result in an increase in the complexity of neural processing involved in eye movement control. Clear typography requires careful adjustment of spacing parameters to avoid ambiguity, and visual displays rarely allow for such adjustment because of the limitations of software and, ultimately, of spatial resolution.

If there is a general increase in the complexity of the neurological processing involved in vision when visual displays are used, discomfort, eye-strain, and headaches may be a consequence. There have been several surveys and reviews (e.g. Dainoff 1982; Evans 1987) reporting an association between visual discomfort and the use of computer displays, although the association is not invariably obtained (Howarth and Istance 1985). It remains to be seen whether, as hypothesized here, these complaints are attributable to pulsating light and the requirement for accurate control of eye movements.

It has been shown in Chapter 6 that the invisible pulsation of light from fluorescent lamps can be responsible for headaches and eye-strain. On a CRT display the pulsation frequency is usually lower than 100 Hz, closer to the frequency at which flicker becomes visible. The variation in luminance with time (modulation) is almost always greater than that from a typical (halophosphate) fluorescent lamp, owing to the use of short-persistence phosphors. Because the flicker is slower and has greater modulation, one might expect it to be more likely to induce headaches and eye-strain, particularly in view of the pronounced effects on eye movement control.

One of the first studies to identify the oscillating luminance of the screen as a problem was a field study by Laubli *et al.* (1983). They measured the variation in luminance of the characters on VDU screens and reported a relationship between the oscillation and a range of complaints. Unfortunately it is difficult to evaluate their findings because of a paucity of technical details.

A subsequent laboratory study compared a cathode ray tube display with a rear-projection display of spatially equivalent material. The continuously illuminated projection displays were preferred (Harwood and Foley 1987).

In the study by Kennedy and Murray (1991) the subjects who showed the greatest impairment of ocular motor control (the skilled typists) were also those who complained of symptoms from VDU use.

7.11 Prevention of discomfort

When using a visual display terminal that pulsates in brightness it may be important to eliminate other sources of light pulsation, such as that from the room lighting. Pulsation from room lighting makes symptoms of discomfort more likely and may, at least in principle, interfere with the pulsation from the VDU screen, being at a different frequency. In Chapter 6 the steps that can be taken to remove pulsation of room lighting were described.

The pulsation of light from computer displays is more difficult to deal with. In general, liquid crystal displays have a lower modulation than cathode ray tubes, but they have poorer spatial resolution, and poorer contrast. Liquid crystal technology is changing rapidly and colour displays are now available. Some have active matrix screens that avoid flicker. These displays are relatively expensive at the moment but will hopefully decrease in price. There are many other types of display, but most exhibit rapid pulsation of light.

In many circumstances there is simply no alternative to cathode ray tube displays. When such displays are unavoidable, long-persistence phosphors can reduce the disruptive effects of light pulsation (Neary and Wilkins 1989). These phosphors are unsuitable for dynamic displays, but may be preferable for static textual material. They are available with green or amber phosphors, and, for reasons described below, amber phosphors may be preferable.

Mesh screens in front of the surface of the cathode ray tube reduce the brightness of the screen but enhance its contrast, maintaining visibility, as described in Section 7.4. Some operators find such screens helpful, presumably because the effects of pulsation depend on the brightness of the light.

Spectacles with a strong rose or reddish brown tint can reduce the pulsation from halophosphate fluorescent lamps and a suitable tint for this purpose has been developed (see Section 6.10). Anecdotally, this tint also reduces eye-strain from cathode-ray-tube displays and it is possible that some low-frequency beat between the lighting and the CRT display is responsible for complaints, and is reduced by the tint (see Section 6.10).

Discomfort results not only from the temporal but also the spatial characteristics of a display. The way in which text is laid out is critical for providing unambiguous information for the saccadic system, as was shown in Chapter 5. It is important to space text adequately, and to avoid clutter from text that is not necessary for the task in hand. Vertically arranged menus may be more difficult to search than those that are horizontal, if the eyes are required to move horizontally, owing to the shearing of vertical contours during horizontal eye movements (see Section 7.6).

In this chapter we have seen that the cathode-ray tubes used in televisions and computer displays emit light intermittently at frequencies that range from 25 to more than 100 Hz and that at frequencies less than about 60 Hz, flicker is capable of inducing eye-strain, headaches, and epileptic seizures in those who are susceptible. At higher frequencies at which the flicker is imperceptible eye-movements are disturbed, and this disturbance may play a rôle in inducing headaches and eye-strain. In the next chapter other more general aspects of the design of our environment are discussed.

8 Design

Our visual environment is full of stripes and they can have harmful and annoying effects. Sometimes they are a deliberate feature of design, but more often they are the result of modular construction.

In Chapters 2 and 3 we have seen that when patterns have particular spatial characteristics they can induce anomalous visual effects, eye-strain, headaches, and even seizures. In this brief chapter we consider first the spatial characteristics of the visual environment that humans have created for themselves. The environment is full of stripes of various kinds, and they can and do have harmful effects. Having considered design in this general context, we turn to design in relation to lighting.

8.1 Stripes are everywhere

The story behind this book began in 1973 when the author was asked to examine a little girl who had pattern-sensitive epilepsy. Every time she looked at patterns of striped lines she suffered a fleeting loss of awareness, an absence seizure. She was sensitive to the stripes from radiators, grills and gratings, patterned clothing, furnishing fabrics, and so forth. Figure 8.1 shows a histogram of the seizure incidence obtained from a continuous 48-h EEG recording. The recording was made using ambulatory equipment that enabled the patient to move around her normal environment. As can be seen, the rate of seizures averaged about 20 per hour – one every three minutes.

Covering one eye can greatly reduce epileptic photosensitivity (Chapter 2). The patient was therefore fitted with a pair of spectacles with one frosted lens in an attempt to see whether her seizures would be reduced. It turned out that the incidence of seizures was reduced by over 90 per cent, to only two per hour. The effect of covering one eye in this way provided evidence that most seizures were the direct result of visual stimulation.

As far as we were able to judge from laboratory investigations, the patient suffered seizures in the waking state *only* when she saw striped patterns, whether they were from radiators or laboratory equipment, or presented as part of an EEG investigation. The rate of seizures suffered by this patient in her normal environment is therefore testimony to the widespread occurrence of stripes in the urban environment.

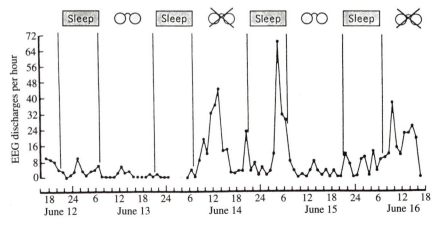

Fig. 8.1 Seizure incidence during a continuous 48-h EEG recording of a patient with pattern-sensitive epilepsy. The recording was made using ambulatory equipment that monitored the EEG while the patient went about her daily activities. (After Ives *et al*. 1976.).

Stripes are indeed a common feature of design, as can be appreciated from Fig. 8.2 which shows a collage of stripes of various kinds. They occur at a wide range of spatial scales – from the exterior of buildings to the furnishings within them.

8.2 Effects of striped designs

The unfortunate reaction of the above patient was extreme and rare. Other less extreme reactions are relatively common, as the following examples show.

1. When metal-treaded escalators were first introduced on the London Underground there were complaints concerning the visual effects that the stair-tread produced. These complaints reached the medical press (Collins 1969).

2. The British Transport and Road Research Laboratory introduced yellow stripes painted across the road surface at the approach to traffic intersections. The spacing of the stripes gradually decreases so as to create an illusion of increasing speed. The illusion has the effect of slowing vehicles, and reducing accidents. The lines can contrast strongly with the road surface on which they are painted, and from certain viewing positions

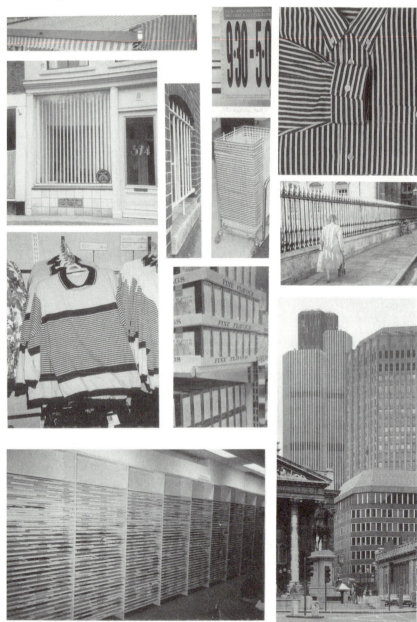

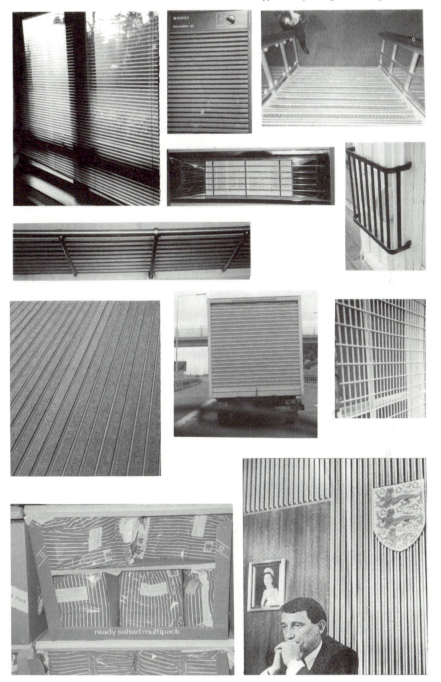

Fig. 8.2 Some stripes in our environment.

can have aversive characteristics. When the stripes were first introduced there were complaints, and the Migraine Trust became involved. Then a letter in the medical press described a man in whom an attack of partial awareness occurred whilst he was driving over the lines. Fortunately, he managed to brake and stop his car without accident. When we recorded an EEG, epileptic photosensitivity was demonstrated.

3. A new coffee bar at the Bristol Royal Infirmary featured zigzag black and white stripes on the floor and a wooden screen in red check. Complaints reached the national press.

4. When the psychiatric unit of Hereford County Hospital was opened there were many complaints concerning a garish carpet that was giving people headaches. These complaints reached the national press. The carpet had a tiled design (tessellation) which, when viewed from a distance, formed a pattern of stripes (see Fig. 8.3), and the stripes had spatial characteristics appropriate for discomfort. The problem was eventually overcome by positioning pot plants so that large areas of the carpet were not simultaneously visible.

5. A small design firm was commissioned to arrange the layout of an office and, for greater privacy, provided partitions between computer workstations. The partitions were decorated with a striped pattern. The stripes had to be removed after the design was commissioned owing to complaints from users and from management.

6. When the artist Bridget Riley held an exhibition of her striped art, the guards complained of headaches and requested dark glasses (Daily Telegraph 1971).

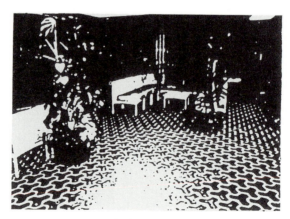

Fig. 8.3 Headache carpet in hospital.

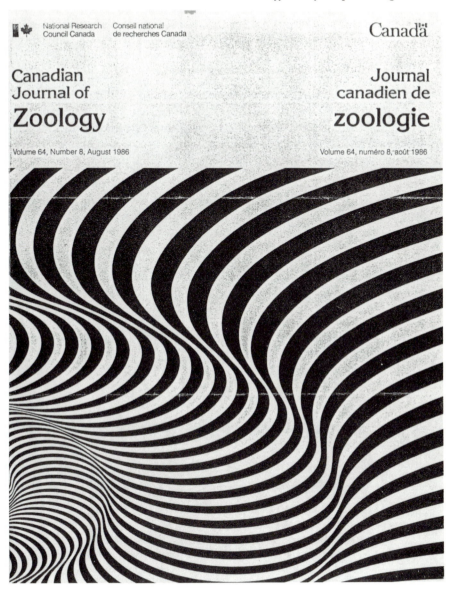

Fig. 8.4 A journal cover that the editor sought to have removed. Courtesy of the editor.

7. A design team was responsible for the new cover of a scientific journal incorporating a striking design of curving stripes, see Fig. 8.4. The editor sought to have it replaced.

8. The advertising standards authority received complaints when an advertisement in the national press featured a pattern of swirling stripes above the caption: 'Some people will have a fit when they see this'. According to a subsequent front-page article in the Observer, the prophecy came true, see Fig. 8.5.

9. Certain designs of wallpaper have been responsible for headaches. The wallpaper in Fig. 8.6 was selected by a sufferer. The design has been altered slightly to avoid litigation! Notice that the pattern is not itself striped but forms stripes when large areas are exposed. Note, too, how

OBSERVER SUNDAY 5 NOVEMBER 1989

Advert banned after readers pass out

id be enough.'
hat the adver-
was due to run
reaks its code.
that 'distress
used in an ad-
ock or attract

believes that
it, which was
iire's self-help
rammes, used
language. 'I
olutely shock-
;A's chairman
text could not
d more clum-

th Yorkshire
ts advertising
Rubicam, ac-
)A's ruling,
th expressed
effect of the

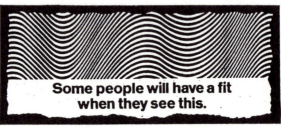

Some people will have a fit when they see this.

Health warning: The prophecy comes true.

'The last thing we wanted to do was cause alarm,' says Yorkshire's controller of corporate affairs Mr Geoff Brownlee. 'In fact my own first reaction when I discussed our agency's planned advertisement was to wonder whether it would cause a fit. But we got assurances that it would not.'

As it happens, the advertisement was written by a copywriter at Y & R, who suffers from epilepsy. The advertisement was also shown in advance to the Epilepsy Association, which could see no particular problems.

Y & R won the £3 million Yorkshire Television account

only three mo
first work has
print and poste
which have tri
Yorkshire Tele
just mean Emm
Last week Y
sion's poster a
the Rik May:
B'stard upset t
York, Mr Con
catchline of tl
'B'stard - In Y
What They Cal
Gregory says t
in very bad ta
work extremel
constituents'.

Yorkshire T
prised at Greg
because it
planned adver
eral Tory MP:
Blackpool part
received no obj

Fig. 8.5 A prophecy that came true. (The stripes in the original advert were larger, covering an entire page of newsprint.) Courtesy of the Observer.

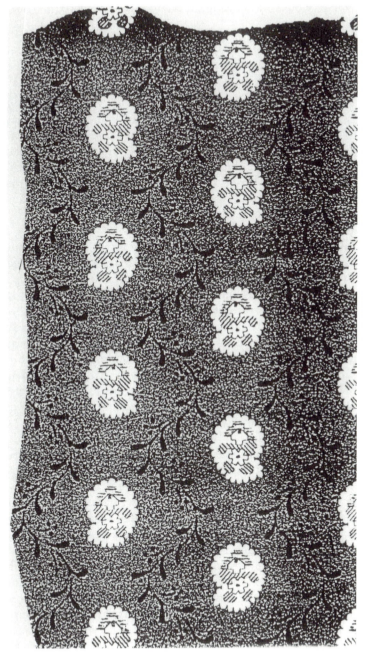

Fig. 8.6 Too much of this wallpaper could cause problems.

difficult it would be to gauge the effects of the pattern from a small sample sheet.

8.3 Deliberate design and modular construction

Noxious patterns can be an intentional aspect of design or an incidental aspect of modular construction. Stripes are sometimes used deliberately to catch the eye. As the frontispiece of this book shows, they can indeed by very striking. There would appear to be a trade-off between the capacity of a visual stimulus to 'strike the eye', and its capacity to 'hit the head'. Unfortunately the nature of this trade-off differs from one individual to another. A pattern that the designer finds attractive may hurt the eyes of the people who have to live with it.

As often as not, stripes result from the way in which construction takes place. Construction is often modular: small parts are pieced together to make a whole. Whether or not stripes result depends on the shape of the parts and the way they are put together: in other words, on the nature of the tessellation. All too often the component parts are identical, and the tessellation has a repetitiveness which at best is boring, and at worst can be quite harmful. The matting used at the entrance to buildings is a case in point. The mat is made from identical sections that alternate ribs of contrasting colours and they provide a pattern with aversive spatial characteristics, see Fig. 8.7. Even patterns with complex tessellations can form stripes when viewed from certain angles. The patterned carpet in Fig. 8.3 is one example; the herringbone cobbles in Fig. 8.8 are another.

Obviously, the tessellation is constrained by the shape of the parts themselves. Bricks, for example, can produce stripes when arranged in the popular herringbone pattern. But it is quite possible to cover a surface with identical shapes in such a way as to avoid stripes. Consider the tessellation shown in Fig. 8.9. The pattern as a whole shows little periodicity, although the basic units of construction are all identical L-shaped brick tiles. Tiles with this shape have the advantage that when large surface areas are tiled in haphazard arrangement no unpleasant visual effects can occur (c.f. the carpet in Fig. 8.3). The tiles are used on the Italian Riviera to provide a floor for beach huts. They are ideal for this purpose because the bright oblique light from the sun accentuates the contours formed by the junctions between tiles. Were the tiles arranged regularly they would have had unpleasant effects. L-shaped tiles are just one of a variety of shapes that will tile a plane surface non-periodically.

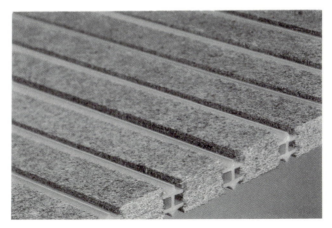

Fig. 8.7 Stripes for wiping your feet on.

8.4 Convenience versus necessity

Only rarely are stripes a necessary aspect of design, although they are often convenient and cheap. The following are examples of stripes that are convenient, but unnecessary.

1. As discussed in Chapter 6, ceilings are often designed with a linear and periodic arrangement of luminaires because it can make wiring simpler. In an open-plan office this arrangement can result in a pattern of very bright stripes in the periphery of the visual field. With a little thought it is quite possible to avoid such an arrangement. On British Rail's Intercity

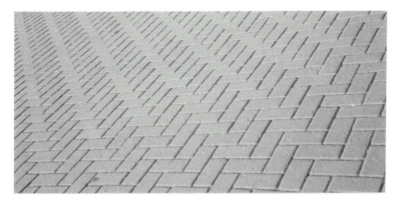

Fig. 8.8 Stripes from cobbles.

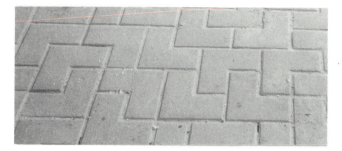

Fig. 8.9 Italian brick floor.

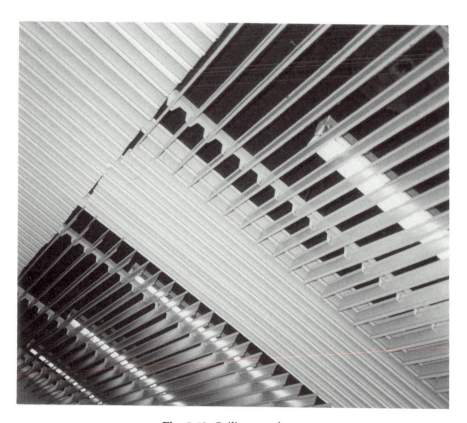

Fig. 8.10 Ceiling panels.

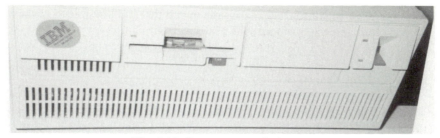

Fig. 8.11 Computer ventilations.

Express the luminaires are arranged to cross the carriage, as shown in Fig. 6.8, rather than to run parallel with it. The result is a pattern of stripes.

2. It is convenient to construct ceiling panels so that they are small and can easily be removed. It is also convenient to be able to see some of the trunking behind the panels. But it is not necessary to design ceiling panels in the form of bars alternating with gaps of equal width (see Fig. 8.10).

3. Ventilation grills on consumer electrical goods are often designed using a ribbed plastic moulding. It is possible to avoid stripes with unpleasant characteristics, and it is certainly not necessary for the grills to be a conspicuous feature of design. Nevertheless grills with unpleasant visual characteristics are placed on the front panels of computers where they are positioned so that they catch the eye of the operator, see Fig. 8.11.

4. It is convenient to design metal treads on escalators with a raised ribbing narrow enough to prevent small objects getting trapped in the comb at the top and bottom[1]. It is not necessary to construct the stair treads in a bright metal. The surface remains bright whilst dirt collects in the space between the ribs, enhancing the contrast of the pattern.

8.5 Natural images

When components in an image are repeated periodically, as in many images from urban scenes, the level of detail changes with scale in an irregular way. Natural scenes have little in the way of periodically repetitive structure. It is scenes such as these that the human visual system evolved to analyse. Natural scenes seem to have the characteristic that at every spatial scale there are few

---

[1] See Safety Code of Elevators Escalators, 1981; American Society of Mechanical Engineers, New York.

configurations of contours that are similar, and that it is possible to confuse. Perhaps human design should take a lesson from nature.

8.6 Lighting design

We now return briefly to the subject matter of Chapter 6 and consider design in relation to lighting.

When a building is commissioned it is necessary to design the lighting system so that the appropriate amount of light will fall on the various surfaces. This involves calculations that take into account the light from a luminaire and the direction in which it is emitted, the reflectances of the surfaces upon which the light will fall, and the position of the eyes of an observer. The Chartered Institution of Building Services Engineers publishes many well-written documents on the subject. Guidance is given to engineers concerning the level of lighting deemed to be sufficient for various types of work. Glare from light reaching the eye from unwanted angles is considered at length, together with techniques for calculating whether a given lighting installation is likely to cause complaints of glare. At present, pattern glare from arrays of ceiling luminaires is not considered.

Just as with other aspects of design, there are trends in lighting design. The trends are motivated by considerations of both fashion and efficiency. Some of these trends are beneficial to health and others are probably detrimental (Wilkins 1992). We will consider some of these trends briefly.

It has become fashionable to use uplighters which direct their light on the ceiling, providing a diffuse illumination. It is necessary to use very bright sources in these lighting schemes and high-pressure gas discharge lamps such as metal-halide and high-pressure sodium lamps are typically used. Chapter 6 identified the 100 Hz pulsation from lighting as causing headaches and eye-strain. The high-pressure discharge lamps cannot yet be operated from high-frequency circuitry and they emit more 100 Hz pulsation than do conventional fluorescent lamps. Their use in office lighting schemes is inadvisable until high-frequency circuitry becomes available.

Another contemporary trend is to replace incandescent lamps with the more expensive, but more efficient, compact fluorescent lamps. Various marketing techniques have been undertaken in Scandinavia to persuade domestic consumers to make the changeover. Many of the early compact fluorescent lamps used conventional circuitry. Fortunately high-frequency ballast is now more common.

The trend towards dimmable ballast is probably good for health and efficiency, provided the ballasts give stable light when dimmed (which is unfortunately not always the case). The ballasts are electronic and operate at high frequency. People like to be able to vary the lighting level to suit themselves, and often choose to work under lighting levels that are lower than would normally be provided, particularly when operating visual display units.

The trend towards narrow (26 mm) diameter fluorescent lamps is unlikely to be detrimental to health. As mentioned in Chapter 6, narrow diameter fluorescent lamps generally show a lower modulation on conventional low-frequency circuitry than the more old-fashioned wide lamps.

In the following chapter we turn from prevention to cure, and consider the role of ophthalmic tints in the reduction of eye-strain and headache.

9   Colour as therapy

A new system for precision ophthalmic tinting is described, together with some preliminary findings.

It should be emphasized at the outset that the subject matter of this chapter is controversial. There have been many claims for treatment using colour that have had little scientific support. Such support has recently emerged, as we shall see, but scepticism will continue to be justified until the research findings have been replicated.

Weston (1962, p. 52) made the observation that:

it is . . . possible for acute (eye) strain to be caused by repetitive patterns . . . For example, a dress fabric having very narrow black and white stripes of equal width – forming what is known as a dazzle pattern – has proved so trying to work with as to be intolerable except for quite short periods. In such cases it is sometimes possible to lessen the strain by wearing coloured glasses which appear to subdue the glaring contrast of the pattern.

In the previous chapters we have confirmed Weston's observation that patterns can be harmful in this way. In this chapter we consider the possibilities for the treatment of pattern-induced glare using coloured glasses.

9.1 Extravagant claims

The use of colour in the treatment of disease has a long history that is itself quite colourful. Many claims have been made with little evidence to support them. Figure 9.1 shows Otto's Improved Light Bath (1901), an apparatus that exposed patients to coloured light: 'the colour of the light can be changed while the patient is in the bath, it being unnecessary for him to leave the same. This is effected by means of providing banks of lamps of various colours, wired so that, by means of a switch lever, the patient can be treated by light of appropriate colour.' One can only hope that no-one died of shock! Later, syntonics became fashionable in the United States. Treatment consisted of sitting before a 'syntonizer' for 20 min periods. The syntonizer provided light with a specific spectral composition. The composition was determined on the basis of syntonic optometric philosophy, that of an 'imbalance in the autonomic nervous system . . . manifest as a sympathetic

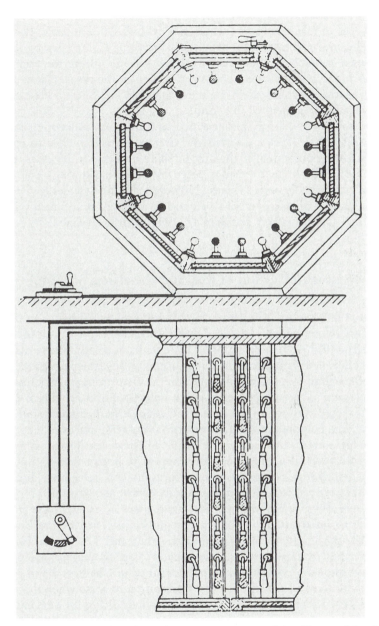

Fig. 9.1 Otto's Improved Light Bath (1901). Courtesy of the Chartered Institution of Building Services Engineers.

or parasympathetic predominance', and giving rise respectively to a tendency of the eyes to turn outwards (exophoria) or inwards (esophoria) (Liberman 1986). In similar vein, a recent pamphlet advertising Color Therapy Eyewear includes a colour reference chart or 'chakra guide' listing the appropriate colours for a variety of body parts: e.g. 'violet for the pineal gland, cerebral cortex, central nervous system, right eye function' etc. There is little evidence for or against treatment of this kind!

An extensive but largely unscientific literature exists concerning colour in sunglasses. Clark (1969) reviewed this literature and was able to conclude that, 'with the exception of therapy in some uncommon illnesses, there is generally no advantage to vision gained by observing through coloured as opposed to neutrally-tinted lenses.' However, coloured glasses have recently been offered as a controversial treatment in dyslexia, amid much publicity. Evans and Drasdo (1991) and Stanley (1991) provide reviews.

9.2 Perceptual distortion of text and the effects of colour

Meares (1980) reported improvements in reading performance in dyslexic individuals when glare was reduced by covering the text with coloured over-lays. Irlen (1983, 1991) also reported benefits from colour. She stressed that many children with a specific reading difficulty describe perceptual distor-tions of text, and that some children think the distortions are experienced by everyone, and so they do not report them unless prompted to do so. The dis-tortions include motion of the letters and changes in their spacing, transient blurring, and coloured halos. The distortions are reminiscent of the illusions reported in patterns of stripes, see Chapter 3. The distortions are often asso-ciated with visual discomfort and they appear to impair reading fluency.

Irlen described a constellation of symptoms and perceptual distortions which she referred to as *scotopic sensitivity syndrome*. The term implies an undue sensitivity of the rod receptors and there is, as yet, little scientific evidence to justify it. However, in recognition of Irlen's contribution, it might be appropriate to refer to the Irlen syndrome. The clinical condition she describes overlaps with certain aspects of photophobia and involves many symptoms of visual discomfort described in Chapters 3 and 5.

The symptoms of the Irlen syndrome reportedly abate when the page of text has a particular colour. The therapeutic colour differs for each individual and can be very specific: slightly different colours having little effect. If Irlen's claims are substantiated, the techniques used until recently by most optometrists to prescribe tinted lenses give patients insufficient choice in the provision of a tint.

Irlen has developed a range of tinted lenses and proprietary techniques for the provision of a specific tint. The tint is custom-made on the basis of an individual's subjective report when comparing a variety of coloured filters placed in front of the eyes, initially singly and then in combinations. Irlen has founded Irlen Centres in several countries, supplying glasses tinted using her techniques. These techniques and the activities of the Irlen Institutes have aroused much interest and controversy. Several potential explanations of the Irlen syndrome have been offered, including placebo effects and conventional optometric problems (Evans and Drasdo 1991).

Wilkins and Neary (1991) examined 20 volunteers with a history of reading difficulty selected by the Irlen Centre in London as having benefited from the use of their tinted glasses. Fourteen were from different families. All had a history of reading problems and only one wore glasses with a refractive correction. Nearly all had good *acuity, contrast sensitivity* and *stereopsis* (in other words they were well able to see small detail and faint contours, and they were able to use differences between the images in the two eyes to form a perception of depth). Ten had poor ocular muscle balance (when the two eyes were not constrained to look at the same object, the axes of the eyes did not remain directed at the same point in space). Problems of ocular muscle balance are common in children with reading difficulty (Evans and Drasdo 1990), and seem to be more common in people with Irlen syndrome (Evans and Drasdo 1991). Seventeen of the 20 subjects had migraine in the family.

Vision with the tinted glasses was compared with vision using (1) dark (*neutral density*) glasses having the same (*photopic*) transmission and (2) untinted lenses that corrected any residual refractive error.

In a few subjects acuity and muscle balance were significantly improved when the tints were worn. For the group as a whole the tints gave a modest increase in the speed of visual search. When subjects were asked to report the illusions they saw in a pattern of stripes, fewer illusions were reported when the tinted glasses were worn, irrespective of whether illusions of colour were included. Nearly all the subjects reported a reduction in headaches when wearing their tints.

Some of the beneficial effects could have been due to changes in motivation, although it is difficult to see how muscle balance could be affected in this way, given that subjects were unaware as to what the test was measuring and how the measurements were made.

One of the disadvantages of this study and other similar studies reviewed by Evans and Drasdo (1991) is that subjects were aware of the colour of the lens placed in front of their eyes before they looked through it and adapted to its colour. It is difficult to obtain a genuine placebo, given that subjects know what perceptual effects are associated with a particular colour. In the next section we describe an *Intuitive Colorimeter* which was designed to overcome some of these problems, and to provide a continuously variable source of coloured light.

9.3 An Intuitive Colorimeter

A wide variety of colours can be produced by mixing three coloured lights in varying amounts, but it can be difficult to mix the lights to match any particular colour. Colours exist in three intuitive dimensions: colour (hue), strength of colour (saturation), and brightness (luminance). All the dimensions change when one of the lights is varied. The way in which the lights interact to produce a given colour is not obvious (for example, yellow is produced by mixing red and green light). It can therefore be difficult and time consuming to mix a particular shade. Burnham (1952) overcame some of these difficulties with a device that enabled colour to be explored without a change in brightness, and Boynton and Nagy (1982) developed Burnham's device in an apparatus that produced chromatic differences suitable for investigating colour blindness. Neither Burnham's apparatus nor that of Boynton and Nagy provided an observer with the opportunity of mixing colours in an intuitive manner, that is, by varying hue, saturation, and brightness independently. We have therefore developed a simple variant of the Burnham colorimeter that enables an observer to change just one dimension at a time. For example, hue can be varied, keeping saturation and luminance more or less constant (Wilkins *et al.* 1992*b*).

Figure 9.2 shows the principle of the colorimeter. A transparent disc is divided into three sectors, each covered with a different filter so as to transmit light of a different colour. For example one sector might transmit long-wavelength light (and be red in colour), one intermediate wavelengths (appearing green), and one short wavelengths (appearing blue). A collimated cylindrical beam of white light passes through the disc, and is coloured as a result. The coloured light is then mixed as it is reflected and scattered from the matt white inner surfaces of a box. Text is mounted on one surface of this box and viewed through an aperture. When the disc is concentric with the beam, the three filters each pass a similar proportion of the light. The spectral characteristics of the filters are adjusted so that the mixed light is a suitable white (e.g. standard daylight, *D65*).

The disc is free to move so that the beam can pass eccentrically through it. The filters then no longer have similar area. The colour of the mixed light becomes progressively deeper and deeper (more and more saturated) as eccentricity increases. The disc is also free to rotate. This changes the colour.

Colour can be represented in terms of the *Uniform Chromaticity Scale* (UCS) diagram of the *Commission Internationale de l'Eclairage* (CIE) (see Fig. 9.3(a)). This UCS diagram shows all the colours at constant luminance. The curved perimeter represents the colours of the spectrum, the ends of which are joined by a line representing purples that are not in the spectrum and that result from mixing various quantities of red and blue light. In general, any two points in the diagram can be joined by a line representing all the colours that can be formed by mixing lights having the colours represented by the two points. The distance between two points in the diagram roughly corresponds to the ease with which their colours can be discriminated.

Figures 9.3(b) and (c) show the colours obtained by rotating the colorimeter disc: they lie on near-circular loci centred on white. Changing the

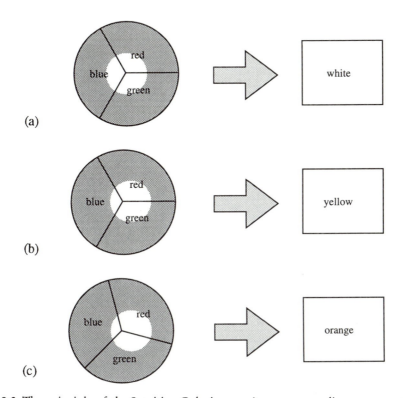

Fig. 9.2 The principle of the Intuitive Colorimeter. A transparent disc represented by the large diameter circle is divided into three sectors bearing a red, green, or blue filter. The disc is free to rotate about a central axis, and the axis can move horizontally varying its position with respect to a stationary circular beam of white light, the centre of which has the same vertical position as the centre of the disc. After passing through the disc, light from the beam is mixed by multiple reflection. (a) When the beam and disc are concentric, rotation of the disc is without effect. The transmission of the filters and their relative angular size can be adjusted so that the mixture has the coordinates of a suitable reference white. (b) As the disc is moved horizontally within the beam, the relative proportions of the three primary colours change. (c) Rotation of the disc changes the colour, and the saturation of the colour varies monotonically with the eccentricity of the disc.

eccentricity of the coloured disc moves the coordinates along radial curves from white.

In the following studies two versions of the above colorimeter have been used. In the initial studies the colorimeter had the gamut shown in Fig. 9.3(b) and in later studies involving precision tinting, the gamut in Fig.

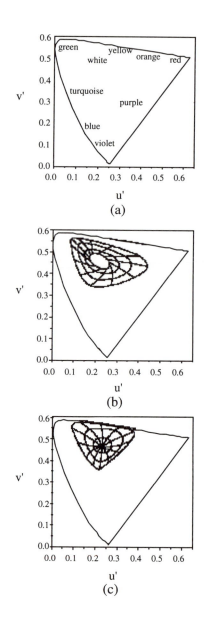

9.3(c). Figure 9.4 shows a cross-section of the apparatus. The mathematics and geometry of the colorimeter are discussed in more detail by Wilkins *et al.* (1992*b*).

The colorimeter had several advantages for research. Not only could hue, saturation, and brightness be varied independently, the variation was continuous rather than discrete; an infinite choice of colour could be made within the range (*gamut*) available. No coloured surfaces were visible within the colorimeter, so it was unnecessary to consider the particular spectral power distribution of the illuminating light, and related *colour constancy mechanisms* (these will be discussed later). The effects of coloured light could be assessed whilst the eyes were adapted to the colour.

9.4 Colorimeter: preliminary findings

Twenty-two children with reading difficulties were examined while the apparatus underwent development. The children were selected as reporting perceptual distortion of text, for example, instability of words or letters (the letters 'wobbled', 'fizzed', 'moved about'). Some of the children were referred by local educational psychologists and teachers, others were brought by their parents in response to an article in Living Magazine which described the perceptual distortions of text that children sometimes report. The children were asked to vary the colour of the light to see whether they could obtain a setting that reduced their perceptual distortions. Settings were obtained at a variety of levels of saturation whilst they observed a page. The page resembled text and consisted of random letters arranged in strings one to seven letters in length (Wilkins *et al.* 1992*b*).

An 18year old girl provided the data shown in Fig. 9.5(a). She was asked to rotate the disc of the colorimeter, varying colour, to see if she

---

Fig. 9.3 (left) (a) The Uniform Chromaticity Scale Diagram of the *Commission Internationale D'Eclairage*, 1976. (The colour names are for guidance only.) The bold curve line indicates the *spectrum locus*, on which lie all the colours of the rainbow and the straight line connecting the ends of the spectrum locus represents non-spectral purple colours. Colour within the surface enclosed by the spectrum locus and the *purple line* can be obtained by mixing lights. The coordinates of the mixed colour (its *chromaticity coordinates*) will lie on a line joining the chromaticity coordinates of the two colours from which it is mixed. (b) and (c) The chromaticity coordinates obtained in the colorimeter. The closed concentric curves show the coordinates obtained as the colour disc is rotated. The radiating curves show the chromaticity coordinates that result when the eccentricity of the disc is varied. (b) shows the values for an early version of the colorimeter, and (c) those for a later version.

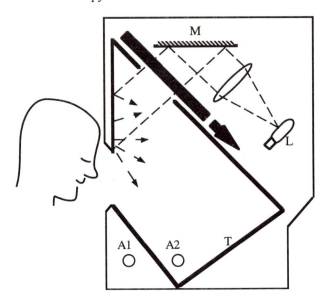

Fig. 9.4 Cross-section of the colorimeter. Light from a collimated source (L) is directed via a mirror (M) through a transparent disc (shown in grey) in which colour filters are sandwiched. The light passes into a box with matt surfaces of high and spectrally even reflectance. The light is scattered within the box, mixing the three colours provided by the disc. The disc can be rotated. It can also slide in the direction shown by the bold arrow. This varies the colour of light incident upon text (T) seen by the observer. A surface lit with white light is visible through port A1 and can be compared with the surface of the text visible through a second port A2.

could find a setting in which the distortions on a page of text disappeared. The settings are shown with the symbol '+'. The subject was then asked to turn the disc slowly until the distortions reappeared, and the settings are shown with the symbol '−'. She did this repeatedly at different eccentricities of the disc. There was a very small area of the chromaticity diagram in which the distortions consistently disappeared. It was so small that it might have been missed by a limited range of tinted glasses.

Data from a 15 year old boy are shown in Fig. 9.5(b). Note that the distortions disappeared when the light was an unsaturated blue or a saturated green. Figures 9.5(c) and (d) represent data from a 10 year old girl obtained on two occasions one week apart.

The technique does not necessarily result in patches in the UCS diagram. It is quite possible for children to report distortions that are inconsistent and may relate to tiredness or other factors. Data for two boys, one aged

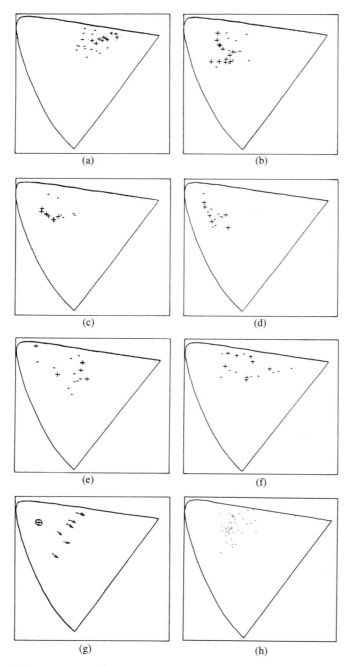

Fig. 9.5 CIE 1976 UCS diagrams summarizing data from children reporting perceptual distortion of text: '-' points show chromaticity at which distortions occurred, '+' chromaticity at which distortions were absent. (a) – (g) show data from individuals and (h) optima from a group of 51 patients.

nine and the other ten, are presented in Figs 9.5(e) and (f) and show an inconsistent scatter in the chromaticity diagram. The data were obtained using the same technique and instructions as those used to obtain the settings shown in the previous figures, in other words the children selected a colour that reduced perceptual distortions, but the reduction was not consistently associated with any particular colour.

Figure 9.5(g) present data for a 14 year old girl who reported a 'pulling in the eyes' when the colour had chromaticity in the lower right-hand side of the CIE 1976 UCS diagram. The setting that maximized comfort is shown by a cross and the limits at which the unpleasant sensation began are shown by the arrows, which also give the direction from which the limits were approached. Note that the limits lie on a line in the UCS diagram. The subject was, of course, quite unaware of the consistency of the settings she was giving.

Figure 9.5(h) represents the optimum settings for a series of 51 patients examined using the colorimeter. Note that the settings are scattered throughout the chromaticity diagram but are more common away from red. The avoidance of shades of red is also seen in adults with migraine when using a colorimeter having gamut similar to that shown in Fig. 9.3(c) (Chronicle and Wilkins 1991). Most of the children had migraine or a family history of migraine. Their tendency to choose colours complementary to red is therefore consistent with the findings in adults with migraine.

The above observations would seem to support the claims of Irlen (1991) that certain children are subject to perceptual distortions of text and that for some children but not others the distortions can disappear when the text has a particular colour. The colour differs from one person to another and yet can be specific and consistent. Preliminary work indicates that the consistency can be close to that obtained in normal observers when they are repeatedly shown a particular shade of colour and asked to reproduce it immediately from memory.

Given that certain observers are able to use the colorimeter to find a colour that improves the clarity and comfort of printed text, the question arises as to whether they would benefit from tinted glasses, and, if so, whether the colour obtained in the colorimeter provides an indication of the appropriate ophthalmic tint. A priori considerations would suggest that the colorimeter setting is not likely to be of use in the selection of such a tint. The brain constructs a 'model' of a light source from the light reflected by a large number of surfaces that differ in the way they scatter and reflect light of different wavelengths. It uses this 'model' to discount the effects of the illuminating light, and compute the colour of the surfaces on the basis of the light they reflect, rather than the colour of the light reaching the surfaces. A pair of tinted lenses has an effect similar (but not equivalent[1]) to that of changing the colour of the illuminating light. Within limits, coloured surfaces viewed through a tinted lens look more or less normal, and the colour of the illuminating light is perceived to have changed.

In brief, the brain takes the colour of the illuminating source into account, and it does so on the basis of light reflected from coloured surfaces. These brain mechanisms enable an object to appear the same colour under a wide range of lighting conditions, so-called *colour constancy* (Land 1977). In the colorimeter, which has only 'white' and 'black' surfaces (surfaces with uniform spectral reflectance) the mechanisms of colour constancy should not necessarily act in the same way as they do when the colour is provided by tinted glasses. This is because, when tinted glasses are worn, a variety of surfaces with different spectral reflectance are visible. The following study suggested that despite the above considerations, the colorimeter setting does in fact provide a good indication of a potentially therapeutic colour for tinted lenses.

9.5 Comparison of techniques

Nine children (aged 12–16) who reported perceptual distortion of text and who had severe reading difficulties were assessed using the colorimeter and also by the alternative proprietary techniques developed by Irlen. As described earlier, these latter techniques involve the repeated application of coloured trial lenses, initially singly and then in combination. Irlen's proprietary examination took place in a room lit by a mixture of daylight and the light from a fluorescent lamp. The order of the examinations was counter-balanced, and they were performed within 2–24 h of each other.

Given the difference in techniques, it was surprising that, in eight of the nine children, the colour appearance of the combination of trial lenses agreed very closely with the colour appearance of the colorimeter (h_{uv} within ± 20 deg). The ninth did not give a consistent setting in the colorimeter. This suggested that in severe cases, at least, the colour setting was robust and that it was relatively unaffected by the presence of coloured surfaces in the field of view. (Coloured surfaces were visible when trial tints were used, but the colorimeter had no coloured surfaces.) Perhaps the mechanisms responsible for the distortions involve visual brain areas previous to those in which constant colours are computed and depend instead simply on the relative activation of the photoreceptors.

---

[1] Some surfaces fluoresce which means that a coloured lens can never have exactly the same effect as a change in the colour of the light sources.

The findings further suggested that the colorimeter could provide a rapid indication of a potentially therapeutic tint. To assess whether this was the case it was necessary to develop a tinting system. This was because many of the settings in the colorimeter could not easily be reproduced with the cosmetic tints available on the market and because the Irlen tints are proprietary.

The colorimeter has the advantage that the effects of coloured light are assessed while the eyes are colour adapted. Adaptation to coloured light can take minutes (Heyhoe and Wenderoth 1991) and any system that relies on an observer comparing coloured trial lenses cannot allow for such adaptation.

9.6 Therapeutic precision tinting: lenses and dyes

Most modern spectacle lenses are made from plastic, usually a resin (allyl-diglycol-carbonate). Lenses made from this resin can be dyed simply by immersing them in hot organic dyes. The molecular matrix expands with the heat allowing molecules of dye to pass into the surface where they are trapped when the lens cools. The temperatures required are about 95 °C and are therefore easily obtained. The dyeing is quick, lasting only minutes. It is also cheap (the dyes cost no more than a few pence per lens). The process has the further advantage that the take-up of dye is independent of the thickness of the material, which is of obvious importance for spectacle lenses. Because the dyes do not interact chemically with one another it is possible to mix them in any proportion and obtain an enormous range of colours.

Wilkins *et al.* (1992*a*) selected dyes on the basis of six principles.

1. Where primary dyes were available, they were used in preference to the composites (mixtures of chemicals) commonly used for cosmetic dyes. Primary dyes were available for all except green, which was provided by mixing turquoise and yellow primary dyes.

2. The dyes were chosen for their stability in the tint bath.

3. The spectral transmission curves of lenses tinted with the dyes were as smooth as possible. With the dyes available for the cosmetic tinting of spectacles the spectral transmissions are sometimes very uneven. When dyes are combined, one transmission curve is multiplied by another, which can increase the unevenness. An uneven spectral power distribution can increase the confusability of one colour with another (increase *metamerism*).

4. The dyes were suitable for rapid tinting. For blue, the dye with the smoothest spectral transmissions was far too slow to be practical.

5. The hue angles of the dye colours were equally spaced, so as to sample colour space evenly.

6. Although it would be possible to use a small number of dyes, a relatively large number (seven) was selected so there would always be one colour from the selection that would have a colour appearance close to that of the colorimeter setting. This simplifies the selection of dyes, as will be seen later. When absorbed by the resin the dyes had the following colour appearances: rose, orange, yellow, green, turquoise, blue, and purple.

The spectral transmission from a dyed lens depends on a large number of factors, particularly the time for which the lens is immersed in the dye, the temperature of the dye bath and the particular quality of the resin from which the lens is made. The latter is difficult to control, and so the tinting procedure needs to make allowance for this variation.

Trial lenses were prepared with different degrees of deposition of dye so as to vary the saturation of colour. The trial lenses were arranged in pairs (one for each eye) and five pairs were provided for five of the seven dyes (but with six pairs for rose and purple). The colours of the five lenses of each dye are shown in the UCS diagram in the central panel of Fig. 9.6. (large points).

The deposition increased geometrically from one pair to the next (see Fig. 9.6, peripheral panels) so that 31 (i.e. $2^5 - 1$) levels of dye deposition could be obtained by superimposing the trial lenses, adding them in all possible combinations.

The trial lenses for two dyes could be combined so that $31 \times 31 = 961$ tints with colours in between those of the two dyes were obtainable. Figure 9.6 shows the chromaticity coordinates of the 961 combinations of orange and rose, the 961 combinations of rose and purple, purple and blue, blue and turquoise, etc. As can be seen, a large area of the UCS diagram has been evenly and densely sampled (6727 points in all) using only two dyes at a time, both with similar hue angle. The area is extended as shown by the broken line when a sixth trial lens is added for the rose and purple dyes. The amount of light transmitted by the tints (photopic transmission) could be separately adjusted by adding lenses dyed using a neutral (grey) dye.

The trial lenses served three purposes:

(1) they provided a colour standard;

(2) they enabled a patient to try out a tint before it was made up;

(3) they facilitated the tinting of spectacle lenses, overcoming the variation in dyeing mentioned earlier.

The Intuitive Colorimeter forms the basis of the tinting system. It is used to assist the patient in obtaining a suitable colour under conditions of

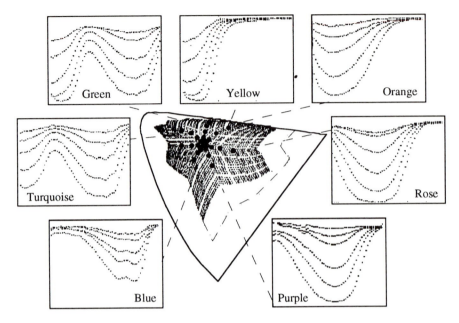

Fig. 9.6 *Centre*: CIE 1976 UCS diagram showing chromaticity coordinates of the trial lenses (large points) and combinations of these lenses (small points) when the dyes were combined two at a time. The broken line shows the outer boundary of coordinates obtainable when a sixth rose lens is added. *Periphery*: Transmissions of the trial lenses (0–100 per cent) as a function of wavelength (400–700 nm). (After Wilkins *et al.* 1992*a*.)

adaptation. This colour is then matched with the trial lenses, and given to the patient to try out. After adjustments to the tint have been made, the patient is given spectacle lenses tinted to the appropriate shade.

9.7 Therapeutic precision tinting: assessment and tinting procedure

The colorimeter contained an A4 page of random letters arranged to resemble text, unless the subject's signs or symptoms suggested that this was too uncomfortable to view, in which case the text was partially covered with white paper.

Beginning with a low saturation, the subject slowly rotated the disc of the colorimeter, varying hue angle, noting the colours that made the text least comfortable. These hue angles were subsequently avoided, particularly at higher saturations. The subject then set the disc to a colour that was the most comfortable. If the subject found this difficult, a colour complementary to the least comfortable colour was chosen by the examiner. Next, the subject varied saturation until the best setting was achieved. The hue angle was then fine-tuned, by instructing the subject to operate the disc 'in much the same way as the dial on a radio set'. If the subject again appeared uncertain, alternative settings of hue and saturation were provided by the examiner for successive pairwise comparison. If consistent settings were not obtained, the procedure was terminated. If consistent settings of hue and saturation were obtained, luminance was varied by interposing different grades of metal mesh in the beam of light so as to assess whether a neutral (grey) tint was necessary.

The following procedure was then used to obtain the combination of trial lenses that matched the colorimeter setting. The viewing aperture was closed, revealing two comparison ports: the first port showing a white surface within the box, lit with the appropriate mixture of coloured light, and the second, a white surface lit with 'cool white' fluorescent light (CIE category F2), luminance 35 cd m^{-2}. The examiner selected a trial lens that was nearest in appearance to the colour of the first port and held this in front of the second so as to compare the colour appearance of the two ports. The examiner then superimposed a trial lens from only one of the neighbouring colours to refine the colour appearance, selecting trial lenses from only two dyes until the colour appearance of the two ports matched. A duplicate combination of lenses was prepared and the two sets of lenses given to the subject to try as a pair (one lens combination for each eye). The subject compared this combination of lenses with combinations of a range of similarly coloured lenses and lens combinations in order to select the one most comfortable for viewing text and natural scenes. In particular, the subject was given the option of reducing the saturation of the colour, and the lowest saturation sufficient to reduce symptoms of discomfort and perceptual distortions was selected.

The chosen trial lenses from one eye were separated into two stacks, each stack consisting of lenses tinted with the same dye. The spectacle lenses were dipped into one dye until the colour appearance matched that of one of the stacks of trial lenses. The trial lenses from the second dye were then added to the stack so that all the relevant trial lenses were now superimposed. The spectacle lenses were then dipped into the second dye until the colour appearance matched that of all the superimposed trial lenses. The colour appearance was judged when the spectacle lenses and the stack of trial lenses were placed side by side on white paper and viewed through two apertures in a sheet of white card, thus eliminating the perceptual effects of the edges of the lenses. The comparison was made under three different types of lighting ('full-spectrum' fluorescent light, tungsten – halogen light, and daylight). When matched in this way, the spectral transmission of the spectacle lenses was virtually identical to that of the stack of trial lenses, differing only slightly in overall transmission. There was little room for error, given that the same dyes were used for the trial tints and the spectacle lenses.

9.8 Therapeutic precision tinting: initial clinical results

9.8.1 Case histories

The following cases have proved particularly instructive.

A 14 year old girl complained of daily headaches behind the right eye, which was amblyopic. Letters appeared unstable: she would read *was* for *saw* and vice versa. She was given yellow glasses after an assessment similar to that described above. She kept a diary from which the following are quotations: 'All stress went from my eyes that I did not know was there ... Can read faster ... Don't need to think hardly ... MUCH easier ... When reading, words spread out. Have realised that is why I used to write with very large spaces between words. Now I don't – that means I don't get told off any more ...' She goes on to describe a reduction of her headaches.

A 20 year old lady had a similar problem, although her reading difficulties were more severe. It had been noted that she was unable to read words correctly because she was uncertain as to the relative position of letters. She would also read *saw* as *was*, *on* as *no*, etc. When she read using a yellow colour, either in the colorimeter or using tinted lenses, the errors of reversal no longer occurred. She reported that the letters did not then move around. She had a early history of strabismus, treated with eye exercises that were not completed. Her acuity in the left eye was poor. Covering one eye improved reading but did not prevent the reversals.

Tinted glasses appear also to have been helpful in four cases of photosensitive epilepsy. The following is one of the clearer cases. A 32 year old lady suffered from photosensitive epilepsy (discussed in Chapter 2). She was intolerant of the antiepileptic drug, *sodium valproate*. She selected a rose tint. 'I find now that bright electric light, whether fluorescent or incandescent, no longer causes discomfort. I can only describe the relief as comparable to a cool breeze in an over-heated environment ... I can now read for quite long periods or watch television without developing the tiredness/headache that was previously so common. I have had no recurrence of epilepsy since using the spectacles ...'

Two cases of severe migraine also appear to have benefited. A 45 year old lady had a 10-year history of classical migraine with several attacks per week. She was admitted to hospital in 1989 with a suspected subarachnoid haemorrhage. The CT scan was negative and the final diagnosis was probable vascular headache. She selected a yellow tint and has suffered only two attacks in the last 6 months, both minor.

A 42 year old lady reported two isolated episodes of loss of left-sided vision without associated pain. Nearly every day she suffered nausea 'like being car sick'. She selected a blue tint. She has had only two episodes in the last 6 months. The remission of symptoms has meant that it has proved possible to withdraw all *propanolol*, a *beta blocker* used to prevent migraine.

One patient with reading difficulty was also subject to attacks of panic. A 43 year old lady suffered panic in supermarkets. She selected a yellow tint. Now she no longer panics, and reports improved balance. She is an artist by profession and when drawing she finds she is no longer reversing shapes.

The history of a 25 year old lady brings all these points together. She had suffered two seizures, and her EEG demonstrated photosensitivity. She suffered one to three bad headaches per month. She reported a barrel-like distortion of a page of text, with words jumping 'in much the same way as stripes do on a striped shirt when you are trying to iron it'. She had discovered for herself that these distortions disappeared when she looked through an orange – brown lens. In the colorimeter she could not find this brown colour but was surprised when the distortions disappeared under an orange – yellow light. Brown is not available in the colorimeter. (It is perceived when a yellow or orange surface appears dark relative to other surfaces, and all surfaces in the colorimeter, apart from the text, have the same reflectance.) When the coloured lens that matched the colorimeter setting was shown to the patient she immediately recognized the colour as the one that helped. Evidently, in her case, at least, the colorimeter adjustments were being made on the basis of symptoms rather than simply preference or prejudice. She compared a range of similarly coloured lenses and rejected all but one, the one that matched the colorimeter setting. Her headache frequency has since been reduced.

9.8.2 Open trial

The above case studies provided the motivation for an open trial of the tinting system. Fifty-five patients with visual discomfort and a range of associated complaints were given glasses tinted according to the above techniques. Forty-five (82 per cent) claimed benefit from the glasses and were still using them more than ten months later: 77 per cent of these reported migraine in the family (Maclachlan *et al.* 1993). Few of the patients had conventional colour vision deficiencies, at least as measured by simple clinical tests. These findings justified a multi-centre placebo-controlled trial.

9.9 Placebo-controlled trial

The colorimeter and tinting system have been used in a placebo-controlled trial in children. The colorimeter procedure was altered slightly. The text of random letters was reduced in size. The subject first compared white light with moderately saturated coloured light, changing colour in even steps round a hue circle. This enabled the examiner to discover the colours that were unpleasant for the subject, without exposing them for long. The subject then adjusted the saturation of the colour that best reduced distortion, as before, and refined the choice of colour at that saturation. These procedures enabled the choice of colour to be made when the subject had been exposed to the coloured light for several minutes, thus allowing for adaptation.

Spectacle lenses were tinted directly from the colorimeter settings without the subject seeing the trial lenses that matched the colorimeter setting. The tinted lenses that gave the selected chromaticity coordinates under conventional lighting had a colour appearance more saturated than one would expect from the appearance of the page in the colorimeter, owing to adaptation and constancy mechanisms. This meant that when subjects received a pair of lenses they were unable to judge from the colour appearance whether or not the lenses provided the appropriate therapeutic colour.

The spectacles were worn for one month (Period A). They were then retinted and returned two weeks later. The retinted pair were worn for a further month (Period B). Two tints were therefore compared one after the other in the same spectacle frames. Subjects did not have the opportunity to compare the colour appearance of the two tints simultaneously but only after an interval of two weeks. The referring optometrist, the patient, and his teacher and parents are unaware as to which tint (that in Period A or in Period B) matched the colorimeter setting. The colorimeter assessments were undertaken at the same time as tests of colour vision. From the patient's point of view they were simply asked to compare two tints.

One pair of tinted lenses (randomly that in Period A or Period B) provided the colour selected in the colorimeter (i.e. a white page illuminated with white fluorescent lighting had matching chromaticity when viewed through the tinted lenses). The other had a similar saturation but a hue differing just sufficiently to allow perceptual distortion to occur. Where possible, the tints were chosen so that both could be described by a similar colour name (e.g. both were a shade of green, a shade of blue, etc.).

Throughout the trial, participants kept a daily record of any episodes of eye-strain or headache, and noted any distortion of text during reading. In addition, they were assessed using different versions of the new (uncoloured) Neale Analysis of Reading Ability

(1) before any spectacles were provided;

(2) during Period A (whilst they were wearing the first tint); and

(3) again during Period B (when the second tint was being worn).

Other than during the assessment of reading, subjects were free to choose whether or not they wore their glasses, provided they kept a note in the diary of when they were worn.

9.9.1 Selection of subjects

The children were selected for admission to the study on the basis that they had used coloured overlays in class and benefited from their use for a period of at least three weeks. The overlays were sheets of coloured transparent plastic that were placed upon a page of text when reading. Most of the children reported eye-strain or headache when reading, and had reading difficulties. The children were referred for a full optometric assessment and those who were found to have an uncorrected refractive error were given glasses with the appropriate refractive correction. Only if the new correction was worn for more than two weeks and did not reduce symptoms were these children entered into the study.

Before receiving the first pair of coloured glasses all entrants underwent an initial examination of reading using the Diagnostic Tutor form of the Neale Analysis of Reading. The lenses and optometric assessments were provided free of charge. The participants were informed that they were free to choose whether to wear the glasses and when to do so.

No ocular pathology was detected and most optometric findings were within normal limits. Forty-two per cent of the participants gave a history of headaches severe enough to be kept off school; and 57 per cent gave a family history of migraine. The incidence of colour vision abnormalities was similar to that expected.

At the second optometric examination 49/52 subjects said that one or both pairs of glasses had helped. 31 subjects preferred the first pair of glasses, 17 the second, and 4 expressed no preference. Overall, 22 subjects preferred the experimental spectacles and 26 preferred the control. 23 subjects 'did not know' which pair matched the original preferred colorimeter setting; 10 thought the experimental glasses were the ones that matched and 11 were of the opposite opinion. Subjects were not able reliably to replicate the appearance of text seen through either pair of glasses when viewing text in the colorimeter and adjusting hue (given the appropriate setting for saturation).

9.9.2 Chromaticities of the lenses

The chromaticities of the experimental lenses are shown by the points in Fig. 9.7. A line joins the chromaticity of the experimental lens (open symbol)

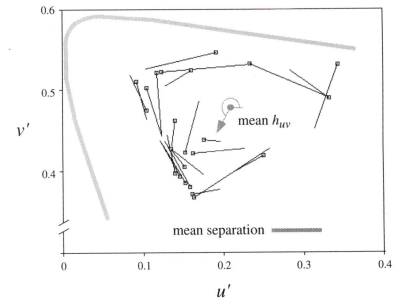

Fig. 9.7 CIE 1975 UCS (u' v') diagram showing the chromaticity of the lenses used in the double-blind trial. Chromaticities of individual subjects' experimental lenses (square points) are connected by a line to the chromaticities of their control lenses. The mean length of the lines represents the average difference in chromaticity between experimental and control lenses and is shown by the grey line in the inset.

with that of the control. Note that, once again, there is a preponderance of lenses with blue and green shades. The average separation of experimental and control lenses is shown by the horizontal grey bar in Fig. 9.7. The separation was small: about six times the just-noticeable difference in colour. The average saturation of the experimental and control lenses did not differ. Both pairs of glasses were worn for a similar period of time: an average of 72 per cent of days for 2.1 hours per day.

9.9.3 Relief of symptoms

Only 36 of the 65 subjects completed their symptom diaries. Days on which the spectacles were worn were divided into those on which headache and eye-strain occurred, and days that were free of these symptoms. Figure 9.8 shows the proportion of days with symptoms when experimental glasses were worn and when control glasses were worn. There are 19 points above the diagonal and 11 below, with 6 at the origin (i.e. showing no symptoms

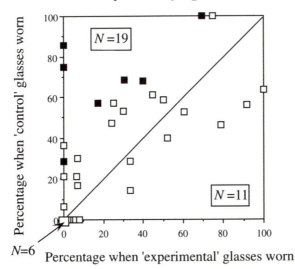

Fig. 9.8 Clinical results of the double-blind trial. Percentage of days when the glasses were worn on which symptoms of eye-strain or headache occurred. Each point represents a subject, and the solid points subjects for whom the difference in symptoms was significant ($p < 0.05$).

with either pair of glasses). The seven solid points indicate the subjects for whom the difference was statistically significant, by individual Fisher's exact tests. For the group as a whole this distribution is most unlikely to have occurred by chance ($p < 0.003$).

The clinical improvements recorded in the headache and eye-strain diaries cannot readily be interpreted in terms of placebo effects. The experimental and control lenses were similar in colour, subjects were not told that one pair was designed to be less effective than the other, and there was always a period of several weeks between the colorimetry and the issue of the first pair of glasses, and between the first and second pair. The double-blind was confirmed by the demonstration that the subjects were unable to distinguish the experimental and control lenses and by their inability to match the colour of either pair of lenses using the colorimeter.

The finding that both pairs were reported to be of benefit, to varying degrees, may suggest that the control and experimental tints were so similar that the subjects were unaware of the slight difference in symptoms with each pair. A more powerful clinical comparison might have been obtained by increasing the chromaticity difference between the two pairs, but this would have weakened the double-blind design. The difference in the chromaticity of experimental and control lenses was small, indicating that the clinically effective tint is idiosyncratic and needs to be determined with precision. The specificity of the therapeutic tint explains the failure of previous attempts to demonstrate the effectiveness of coloured glasses (e.g. Menacker *et al.* 1993) despite anecdotal report of success. Evidently the Intuitive Colorimeter provides one way of determining a therapeutic tint and has the advantage that the effects of the tint can be assessed rapidly while the eyes are colour adapted.

Further studies with larger sample sizes will be needed to confirm the findings of this initial double-blind study. Limited though it may be, the study raises the exciting possibility that we may have new therapy for light sensitivity, and one that may offer benefit not only in children with reading difficulty, but those with migraine. As we will see, the benefit may extend to photosensitive epilepsy.

9.10 Open trials in photosensitive epilepsy

Over the years there have been several published case reports of patients with photosensitive epilepsy who have benefited from coloured glasses. These reports have often included investigations of the effect of coloured flicker on the photoconvulsive response. The latter investigations have often been poorly controlled and in general do not show a consistent effect, see Chapter 2. Newmark and Penry (1979) conclude 'the findings of six studies showed no consistent response . . ., although individual patients may have had an increased sensitivity to one hue or another.' In Jeavons and Harding's (1975) investigation of 17 patients, five showed some increase in sensitivity to red, and the group as a whole showed less sensitivity to blue. The failure to show a consistent or substantial reduction in the response to intermittent light when the light has various colours cannot be taken to suggest that tinted glasses are likely to be ineffectual. As we have seen, seizures can be provoked by patterns as well as flicker, and there have been few studies of the effects of colour on the response to pattern. Indeed the general inconsistency of the response to colour, with a tendency to greater provocation from red is entirely consistent with the findings reviewed earlier in this chapter.

Carterette and Symmes (1952) reported two patients whose seizures were controlled without medication with the use of glasses that absorbed the red end of the spectrum. Their findings were followed by reports from Marshall *et al.* (1953), Courjon (1955), Van Buskirk *et al.* (1959), and Livingston (1972) who reported similar success. More recently Takahashi and Tsukahara (1992) have also reported good clinical results with blue sunglasses. The treatment has not, however, found its way into routine clinical practice.

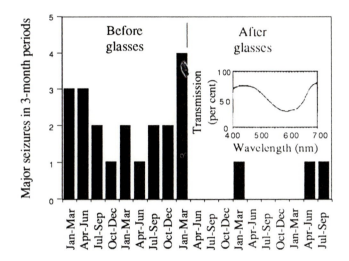

Fig. 9.9 Incidence of major seizures in a 17 year old girl with photosensitive epilepsy before and after blue glasses were provided. The transmission of the glasses is shown in the inset. There was no change in medication throughout the period shown. The incidence of seizures is recorded in consecutive three-month periods.

The author has instigated an open trial of the precision tinting system in patients with photosensitive epilepsy, in view of the medical literature and because of the success in the case histories described above. The subjective methods used with patients with reading difficulty and migraine have been employed once again, although, for safety, the assessment has been conducted whilst the EEG has been monitored. So far, 11 patients have been followed for at least 10 months. Of these, seven are still wearing the tints. In many it is difficult to assess the benefit due to concurrent changes in medication, but Fig. 9.9 shows the seizure record in a patient in whom no changes in medication took place over a 57-month period. As can be seen, the reduction in seizures was considerable, and was maintained. In this patient the tint was blue, but apparent success has also been obtained with other colours, including red. These patients have been adults with epilepsy. Children with epilepsy have been difficult to examine using the subjective methods.

Two patients have been assessed with intermittent photic stimulation. When wearing the selected tint the photoconvulsive response has been reduced or eliminated, but not when wearing grey lenses of similar transmittance. One further patient was examined with patterns, and a similar selective attenuation of the epileptiform EEG response occurred with the chosen tints.

9.11 Overlays

The Irlen Centres supply seven sheets of differently coloured plastic sheets (overlays). These overlays are used in the classroom to select children who might benefit from the use of coloured lenses. The overlays are placed over a page of text in turn, and pairwise combinations compared side-by-side. The child selects the overlay that best reduces the distortion by a process of successive elimination. Sometimes the chosen overlay appears to allow the child to read more fluently and without discomfort.

To date, the literature on the effectiveness of overlays in improving reading is controversial (Rosner and Rosner 1987) and equivocal (Saint-John and White 1988; O'Connor *et al.* 1990; Evans and Drasdo 1991; Stanley 1991; Williams *et al.* 1992). In one of the few placebo-controlled studies, Tyrrell *et al.* (1994) included an untinted transparent overlay with the seven coloured Irlen overlays. They compared the reading and visual search performance of children who selected the clear transparent overlay and those who selected a coloured overlay. Children who selected coloured overlays were more likely to be poor readers. When they read for 15 min with a clear overlay their reading speed decreased slightly but significantly and they reported symptoms of visual discomfort. When, on a different occasion, the same children read using the coloured overlay of their choice, the reading speed was maintained and the symptoms did not occur. Visual search performance was improved. Children who selected the transparent overlay did not show a decline in reading speed, and they reported fewer symptoms of discomfort. The transparent overlay had no effect on their reading or visual search. The above findings suggest that the use of coloured overlays may be associated with a reduction in visual discomfort, with possible benefit for reading.

When colour is provided by lighting or by tinted glasses, the shade people find most helpful varies from one individual to another, and, as we have seen, the colour needs to be quite specific. When colour is provided by an overlay, one might expect the optimal colours to be at least as constrained.

The Irlen overlays are well designed for classroom use: unlike other readily available filters, such as theatre filters, they have a matt coating to reduce specular reflections and they are sufficiently robust to survive the classroom. Unfortunately the range of available colours does not include a purple, as can be seen from Fig. 9.10 which shows the chromaticities of the overlays (large points), and of pairs of overlays superimposed (small points).

An alternative set of overlays has therefore been developed with the chromaticities shown in Fig. 9.11 (Wilkins 1994). The set includes a grey and purple. The overlays are robust and have a non-reflective surface. It is

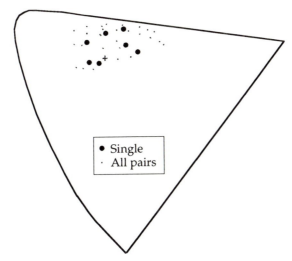

Fig. 9.10 CIE 1975 UCS (u' v') diagram showing the chromaticity coordinates of the Irlen overlays (large points) and of all pairwise combinations (small points). The chromaticity of equal energy white is also shown (+).

possible to combine them two at a time in an intuitive way to provide a wide range of chromaticities. Figure 9.12 shows the chromaticities obtained by superimposing one overlay on another of similar or identical shade. Note that when overlays having neighbouring chromaticities are combined, the chromaticity is not appreciably affected by which overlay is uppermost. The resulting pair of overlays has a chromaticity mid-way between the chromaticity of the component overlays (although the transmission is necessarily lower than that of either individually). This restriction on the combination of overlays to those of neighbouring chromaticity makes the colour mixing intuitive: had other combinations of overlays been used, the resultant colour and transmission would not have been so predictable. For example, if rose and mint-green were combined, the result would have been grey.

The overlays are proving popular, and scientific evaluation is underway.

9.12 A physiological basis for the benefits of coloured tints?

In view of the findings reported earlier in this book, it is now possible to provide a speculative but parsimonious account of the efficacy of tinted glasses in dyslexia, migraine, and epilepsy. We will present the argument step by step together with the inferences drawn from each item of evidence.

1. In patients with photosensitive epilepsy there is considerable convergent evidence that seizures can be triggered in the visual cortex (see Section 2.3).

2. The seizures can sometimes be provoked by patterns of stripes, and sometimes only by stripes in a limited range of orientations (see Section 2.2). *Inference: The trigger can be quite focal in the visual cortex, involving a small hyperexcitable area with columns of cells having the appropriate orientation specificity.*

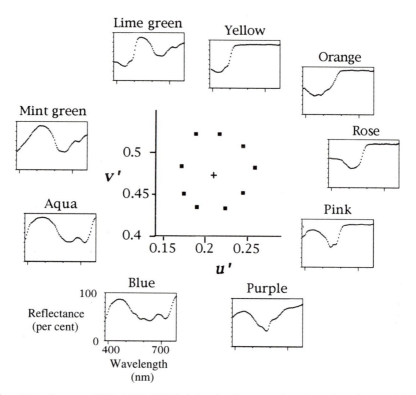

Fig. 9.11 *Centre*: CIE 1975 UCS (*u′ v′*) diagram showing the chromaticity coordinates of the nine coloured overlays (■) and that of equal energy white (+). *Perimeter*: panels show the reflectance (0–100 per cent) of each overlay as a function of wavelength (380–780 nm). The panels are disposed in a manner similar to that of the corresponding chromaticity coordinate.

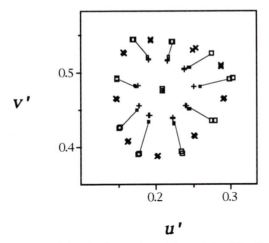

Fig. 9.12 Chromaticities of the single overlays (■) are joined by lines to the chromaticities of two superimposed overlays of the same colour (□). The chromaticities of a single and double grey overlay are shown by the central points. Combinations of a single overlay with a grey overlay (+) and with an overlay of neighbouring chromaticity (✕) are also shown. In every case data for 45/0 and 0/45 CIE reflectance standards are both plotted, but the chromaticities are so similar that the points are almost superimposed.

3. The visual stimuli that trigger seizures in patients with photosensitive epilepsy provoke in others feelings of discomfort and anomalous perceptual distortions (see Chapter 3). *Inference: some of the perceptual effects are due to a spread of excitation in the visual cortex sufficient to excite neurons inappropriately, but not sufficient to provoke a seizure.*

4. People with migraine or with migraine in the family are particularly susceptible to the perceptual distortions seen in epileptogenic visual stimuli. In individuals with consistently lateralized visual aura the distortions are similarly lateralized (see Chapter 3). *Inference: In these individuals the visual cortex of one or both hemispheres may be unusually excitable, but not sufficiently so for seizures to occur.*

5. Text has spatial characteristics that resemble those of stressful patterns (see Chapter 5).

6. Reading can provoke anomalous visual effects, headaches, and photosensitive epilepsy (see Chapter 5).

7. Covering the lines that are not being read, leaving only three visible lines, reduces these adverse effects (see Chapter 5). *Inference: certain*

spatial characteristics of text make reading stressful, particularly for individuals with cortical hyperexcitability.

8. Some cortical neurons are tuned for wavelength or for colour appearance. Others show a less specific response to light of different wavelengths, but none is indifferent to the spectral power distribution of the stimulating light. *Inference: the colour of the illuminating light changes the pattern of excitation in the cortical network.*

9. People with migraine show a consistency not shown by age and sex matched controls regarding their choice of coloured light for reading: they tend to avoid red illumination (see Sections 4.2 and 9.4).

10. Certain children report a reduction in distortion with certain coloured light, different for each individual, but with a tendency to avoid red (see earlier sections of this chapter).

11. These children usually have migraine in the family and suffer frequent headaches (see earlier sections of this chapter).

12. There are case studies reporting success in the use of coloured glasses to reduce seizures in patients with photosensitive epilepsy (see Chapter 2 and above), usually glasses that absorb light at the red end of the spectrum (and therefore appear blue).

13. Precision Tints (selected according to routine subjective methods) reduce the photoconvulsive EEG response to flickering light and patterns (see previous section).

14. Precision Tints also reduce seizures in some patients (see previous section). *Inference: the colour that is therapeutic changes the pattern of excitation in the cortical network so as to avoid local areas of hyperexcitability.*

In the next chapter it is argued that the aversive response to visual stimulation may be due more to activity in the magnocellular pathways than parvocellular, and that activity in magnocellular pathways is reduced by lenses that absorb red light. The arguments are more speculative than the above and therefore appear in a chapter of their own.

10 Speculation

In Chapter 4 we saw that 'strong' visual stimulation can give rise to discomfort and seizures, and at the end of Chapter 9 these ideas were developed into a parsimonious explanation of the effects of coloured glasses in therapy. In this chapter we take these ideas further, but in a frankly speculative manner. We do so from two different levels of interpretation.

10.1 Visual physiology

10.1.1 Excitatory connections between columns

Neurons in the visual cortex are selective for the orientaton of contours in appropriate regions of the visual field, and those with a given preferred orientation are arranged in 'columns' running perpendicular to cortical laminae A complete sequence of preferred orientations occupies about 1 mm (Hubel 1988). The selectivity was originally thought to arise from convergence of excitation of the lateral geniculate nucleus along a line in the visual field. More recently a host of studies employing a variety of techniques have suggested that the orientation selectivity can be attributed to inhibitory connections between cells with different orientation tuning (see, for example, Sillito 1979; Tsumoto *et al.* 1978; Hata *et al.* 1988; Vidyasagar and Mueller 1994). However, there is still considerable debate concerning the relative contribution of excitatory and inhibitory mechanisms to the orientation selectivity. Intracellular recordings seem to show that both the excitatory and inhibitory inputs to a cortical cell are tuned to the same orientation (Ferster 1986). Nevertheless it is possible that, by stimulating only one orientation, a grating compromises intracortical inhibition in some way. The resultant excitation is, after all, concentrated within orientation columns. Long horizontal processes extend laterally from column to column (Gilbert and Wiesel 1983, 1989) and these connections are made only between columns that have similar orientation preference. The connections are excitatory. It becomes difficult to understand why such excitation does not lead to saturated firing of the whole visual cortex! 'Most models of cortical selectivity unsuspectingly run the gauntlet between complete suppression of maximal excitation and a catastrophic breakthrough discharge . . . Our theoretical work shows that strong excitatory transients are very difficult to suppress, unless the magnitude of inhibition is very large indeed.' (Berman *et al.* 1992, p. 449). Meldrum and Wilkins (1984) proposed a minimal and diffuse insufficiency of GABA-ergic inhibition to explain photosensitive epilepsy in man and the photosensitive baboon, *Papio papio*, supported by the pharmacological evidence; the notion being that the insufficiency would manifest itself, given strong excitation, owing to the sharing of inhibitory interneurons between pyramidal neurons. But the issue is far from settled . . .

10.1.2 The magnocellular and parvocellular pathways

Livingstone and Hubel (1987, 1988) have emphasized the separation of two major visual pathways from the retina to the cortex: the magnocellular system and parvocellular system. Within each system the cells have different functional characteristics and are responsible for separate but interconnected streams of information. The pathways take their name from the layers of the lateral geniculate nucleus: two layers with large cells and four with small. The properties of cells in the two pathways appear to differ in four important respects; colour, acuity, speed, and contrast sensitivity.

The cells in the parvo system are coded for colour. Within the geniculate, at least, the majority of parvocellular neurones are 'colour-opponent',[1] responding preferentially to certain wavelengths of light at the centre of the receptive field (long wavelength light in the example shown in Fig. 10.1(a)), and inhibited over a larger region by light of a different range of wavelengths (medium wavelengths in the example). The magnocellular geniculate neurones do not show this opponency but respond to light of all visible wavelengths, although the response may be greater in a certain range.

Within the cortex, the magno cells have a low spatial resolution. They have receptive field centres that are two or three times larger than those of the parvo cells, although all cells have receptive fields that increase in size similarly with eccentricity.

Cells in the magnocellular pathways respond faster and more transiently than parvo cells. They are sensitive to the direction of motion of contours across their receptive fields. They are stereotuned in the sense that they respond to contours in corresponding positions in each eye provided a certain disparity is present. They are more sensitive to low contrasts, but at high contrasts they saturate.

Figure 10.2 shows the magno- and parvocellular pathways in diagrammatic form, together with a summary of their function. Cells in the magnocellular geniculate layers project to layer 4Cα of the striate cortex (visual area 1). This

---

[1]The cells are not strictly 'colour opponent' because they respond to wavelength differences rather than colour (Zeki 1985).

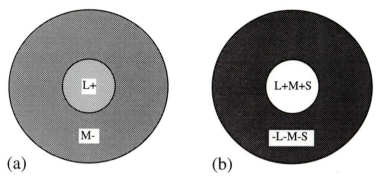

Fig. 10.1 Examples of cells with colour-opponent receptive fields. (After Livingstone and Hubel 1988.)

in turn projects to layer 4B, thence to visual area 2 (V2) and a visual area in the temporal lobe, area MT. Parvo cells project to layer 4Cβ and from there to layers 2 and 3 and thence to V2.

The segregation of information processing seems to be perpetuated in visual areas beyond the visual cortex. Areas in the temporal-occipital region are necessary for learning to identify objects by their appearance, and areas in the parieto-occipital region are needed for tasks involving the positions of objects. Mishkin and Ungerleider (1983) refer to this division as 'what' versus 'where'. The 'what' system may represent the continuation of the parvocellular system and the 'where' system the magnocellular (Livingstone and Hubel 1988).

The properties of the cells in the magnocellular system are therefore reminiscent of those of stimuli responsible for aversive effects. Assembling the points discussed in Chapters 2 and 3, patterns of stripes that differ in colour contrast but not in brightness are not epileptogenic (see Section 2.2.2). The effects of pattern motion (see Section 2.3.5) suggest that directionally sensitive neurones are involved in seizure induction. The effects of binocular fusion (see Section 2.3.1) would be consistent with the action of disparity-tuned neurones. The low spatial resolution of cells in the magnocellular system would be consistent with the spatial frequencies at which aversive effects occur. Similarly, the high temporal resolution would be consistent with the effects of flicker. Epileptiform EEG activity in response to patterns is usually seen over P3 and P4 electrodes (Darby *et al.* 1986), which record from parieto-occipital cortex. Given the work by Mishkin and Ungerleider (1983), the magnocellular system is once again implicated. Magnocellular neurones are more sensitive than parvocellular to contrast across their receptive fields, but they saturate at lower contrasts (about 15 per cent). There is some suggestion of a saturation in the curves

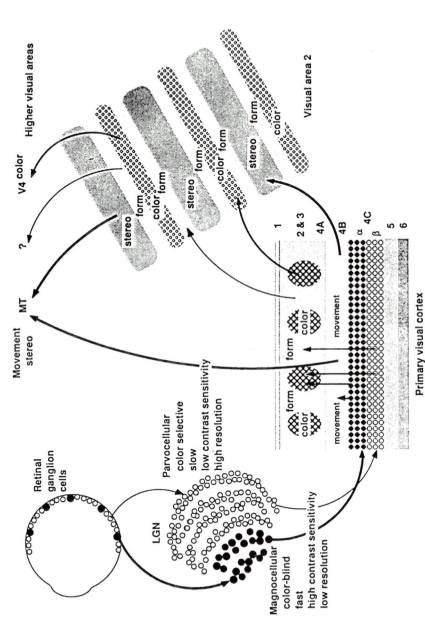

Fig. 10.2 The functional segregation of the primate visual system, showing the lateral geniculate nucleus (LGN), the layers of the primary visual cortex, visual area 2 (V2), and the projections to other areas. (Reproduced with permission from Livingstone and Hubel (1988)).

relating the probability of epileptiform activity to pattern contrast, but not in the corresponding function for illusions (Fig. 3.1).

There is increasing evidence for a selective impairment of magnocellular function in children with reading difficulty. These children perform normally on visual tests thought to be related to parvocellular function, but show deficits on tasks such as flicker perception that are thought to be subserved by magnocellular pathways (Lovegrove *et al.* 1986). The selective magnocellular abnormalities revealed at autopsy in the brains of adult dyslexics are therefore consistent with such dysfunction (Livingstone *et al.* 1991). It is not yet known whether these findings are *specific* to dyslexia, that is, whether similar psychophysical deficits and anatomical changes can be seen in patients with problems other than dyslexia, such as migraine, for example.

Notwithstanding the above pointers towards a predominant role for the magnocellular system, it is difficult to disprove the 'minimal' hypothesis that discomfort is the end product of a non-specific process that results from an excess of neuronal activity in any visual pathway. Further, the distinction between the magno-and parvo-systems has been criticized by Martin (1992) because it takes little account of the information hidden in the 'combinatorial possibilities' of a network of cells. It is the total excitation within this network that is probably the key to the aversive effects of visual stimulation.

10.1.3 Migraine and metabolic demand

People with migraine show deficits in contrast sensitivity that are greater the longer the duration of the disease (see Section 3.6). These deficits suggest that repeated attacks of migraine may damage the visual system. Since migraine affects the circulation of blood in the brain, the visual deficits may result from a transient insufficiency of blood supply. This might be expected to have a greater effect on cells with a high metabolic turnover. There are blob-like regions of layers 2 and 3 of the primary visual cortex of monkeys that are labelled preferentially with radioactive 2-deoxyglucose because of their heightened metabolic activity (Horton and Hubel 1981; Humphrey and Hendrickson 1983). These blobs are also revealed by cytochrome oxidase staining. They receive inputs from both magnocellular and parvocellular pathways. Within the blobs the cells show poor orientation tuning but a colour opponency (Livingstone and Hubel 1988). The surrounding inter-blob cells show no colour opponency. The blob cells project to striped areas of V2 that are also concerned with the processing of colour. Perhaps this is one mechanism for the selective colour preferences shown by people with migraine (Chronicle and Wilkins 1991).

10.1.4 Pain as a response to visual stimuli

The processing of a strong sensory signal is likely to lead to a great deal of neuronal activity. This activity will have metabolic demands that may well be associated with increased regional cerebral blood flow (see Section 4.3). In migraine the mechanisms that tailor the supply of blood to meet metabolic demand may not function as they should, and they may be further compromised by a 'massive' excitation. It is therefore possible that visual stimuli trigger pain by a neurovascular mechanism similar to that in migraine. It is uncertain whether the pain of migraine results from structures within the brain or from vasculature on the scalp or both. The meninges that overlies the cortex is one of the few structures within the brain that is sensitive to pain. Electrical stimulation of the brain surface over the visual cortex during brain surgery results in pain referred behind the eyes (via a branch of the trigeminal nerve), and down the neck via the third cervical nerve, sites where visual display unit operators frequently complain of pain. However, pain can be referred to the eyes from several other intra-cranial sites (Wolff 1963).

It is possible that epileptogenic patterns influence blood flow differently in different individuals. The author (who does not suffer migraine) and a medical colleague who had suffered occasional attacks of migraine with aura collaborated in the following pilot study. We observed an epileptogenic pattern occupying one lateral visual field for five minutes. Cerebral blood flow was monitored following intravenous injection of a radioisotope using two scintillation counters placed over the left and right occipital poles. There was no change in blood flow for the author, but his colleague suffered a headache, and there was a 70 per cent increase in blood flow over the contralateral hemisphere. The findings are merely suggestive, but would be worth replicating, perhaps using less invasive techniques such as transcranial doppler ultrasound, known to be responsive to visual stimulation (Njemanze *et al.* 1992).

10.2 Computational vision

10.2.1 Grouping of the image

The figure of radiating lines (Fig. 10.3) was used by MacKay (1961) to demonstrate some of the illusions commonly seen in patterns of stripes. Do not look at this pattern if you have migraine or photosensitive epilepsy because it might cause an attack. Shadowy arcs are seen at right angles to the lines. These may be related to the diamond shapes (rhomboid lattice) sometimes seen after prolonged observation of patterns of stripes such as the frontispiece. Geometric patterns of lines are *redundant*, in the sense that one part of the image is highly predictable from another. Why should such redundancy give problems for the visual system? Information theory states that redundancy reduces the effects of noise. One might therefore expect predictable stimuli such as the ray figure to be relatively easy to process. We will consider the algorithms that have been proposed for the early stages of vision and show why these stimuli may, in principle, be difficult to process.

David Marr (1982) analysed the information processing involved in vision much as would a computer programmer who wished to make a computer see. There are many computational tasks involved in seeing, and one of the more basic is the detection of those parts of the image where the luminance changes. Marr proposed that a luminance 'edge', or contour, could be detected by computing the *rate* at which luminance changes across space and by noting the point where the rate of change was maximal.

Watt and Morgan (1985) extended these ideas, adopting different mechanisms for contour detection. They emphasized that the image was analysed at a variety of spatial scales. Figure 10.4 shows an example. Information

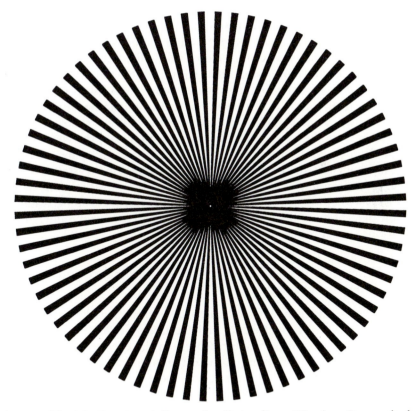

Fig. 10.3 The MacKay (1961) figure of radiating lines. Warning: Do not look at this pattern if you have migraine or photosensitive epilepsy because it might cause an attack.

about details of the image is provided by contours in the high-pass (high spatial frequency) image (Fig. 10.4(b)). Information about the position of these details was obtained from the way they nest within the contours in the low-pass (low spatial frequency) image, see Fig. 10.4(c).

Images such as text and gratings differ from natural scenes in that the low-pass image contains many similar maxima and minima and a confusion of similar contours (see Fig. 5.5(b) and (c)). This might mean that the positioning of the details from the high-pass image is more complex than for other more natural scenes.

As an example of the effects of the grouping that occurs from low-spatial frequency information, consider the image of a piano keyboard. The white keys form a repetitive pattern. If the lid is partially closed so that only the white keys are visible, it is impossible to group the keys. It is also difficult to identify the position of any one particular key, such as middle C. The spatial filters that resolve the individual keys give an ambiguous output because one key is very much like another. The black keys differ from the white keys in that they can be grouped unambiguously. Although the black keys have a repetitive structure, the structure differs at a variety of spatial scales. The structure of the finer scales that resolve the individual keys differs from the structure of the coarser scales that fail to resolve the keys, but resolve instead only the gaps between the groups of two or three keys. Nesting of the information from one spatial scale within that from another is possible.

When the white and black keys are seen together, the low spatial frequency information from the black keys disambiguates that from the white keys. It enables them to be grouped, and as a result of that grouping, individual keys can be identified. It might be argued that the visual system performs an analogous grouping of an image. Images such as gratings are rather like the white keys without the black: they thwart the attempt at grouping, leading to unstable perception as the visual system attempts to resolve the ambiguity at the various spatial scales.

10.2.2 Efficiency of signal transmission on luminance and colour-difference channels

In a completely independent application of information theory to vision, it has been argued by Buchsbaum and Gottschalk (1983) and Moorhead (1985) that signals from the photoreceptors in the eyes are combined into a luminance channel, conveying most of the information, and two colour difference channels, one red – green and the other yellow – blue. They derive this familiar conception from first principles simply by assuming that the transmission of information over visual pathways is made as efficient as possible. They argue that because the receptor spectral sensitivities overlap, it would be inefficient to transmit signals from the receptors directly because

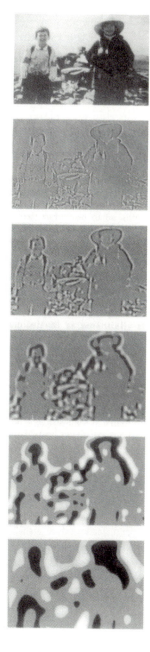

Fig. 10.4 Filtered images. Mexican hat filters (see fig. 5.6) of increasing spatial scale have been applied to the image shown at the top. Reproduced with permission from Watt (1991), Fig. 17, p. 82.

much of the information from one receptor would be shared by the others. Some pre-processing of the receptor output is necessary to reduce the redundancy. The transmission can be made efficient by decorrelating the receptor output and transmitting a luminance signal (the sum of the signals from the three types of cone) and two colour-difference signals (derived from differences in the output of combinations of cones).[2] The visual system does indeed appear to function in this way (Derrico and Buchsbaum 1991). It is perhaps unsurprising that the brain may use optimally efficient signal processing, but it follows from the mathematics presented by Buchsbaum and Gottshalk that if one of the channels were selectively impaired by disease, the information transmission could be re-optimized by changing the relative output from the photoreceptors. Such a change could, for example, result from the wearing of tinted glasses, particularly if the lenses were strongly coloured and overcame the effects of the receptor adaptation.

Given the assumptions made by Buchsbaum and Gottschalk, it is possible to calculate for each colour of lens what the relative energy on the three channels would be, *given optimally efficient transmission*. The calculations need to be taken with a big pinch of salt, given the controversial assumptions that they depend upon. Nevertheless they provide one way of explaining the preponderance of blue tints. The results of the calculations are shown in Fig. 10.5 (Ian Nimmo-Smith, personal communication). In Fig. 10.5(a) the contours show the amount of information (energy) that would be transmitted on the luminance channel, given a lens with a particular colour, the colour of the lens being represented by its chromaticity coordinates in the UCS diagram. The lens is assumed simply to change the relative weights of the long- medium- and short-wavelength cone receptors, L, M, and S, and no allowance has been made for adaptation. (The spectral sensitivities have been calculated from the equations given by Hunt (1991).) The contours are shown relative to the information with no lens, so the contour marked '0' passes through the coordinates of equal energy white. The contours are numbered according to the information in bits relative to no lens: the contour marked -0.1, for example, indicates that $\log_2$ (energy with lens) $- \log_2$ (energy with no lens) $= -0.1$. In other words, if the luminance channel had been damaged, it would be more efficient to distribute less information on the luminance channel and more on the colour difference channels. Figure 10.5(a) indicates that this would be achieved with a blue lens. As can be seen from Figs 10.5(b) and (c), a blue lens will increase the information carried by the colour opponent channels, but the increase on the first colour opponent channel $(L-M)$ will be less than that on the second $(L+M-S)$ channel (both measured relative to the normal conditions with no lens).

---

[2]This is the method used for transmission of colour television signals in the American system (Buchsbaum 1987).

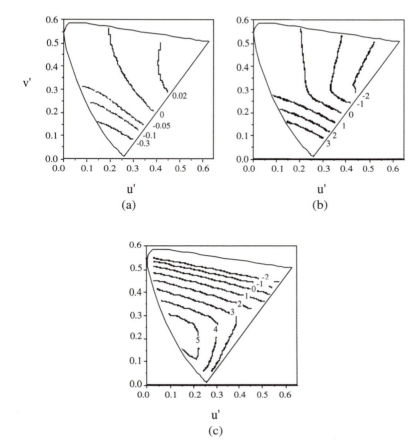

Fig. 10.5 Contours showing the colours giving similar energy in (a) the luminance channel, (b) the first colour opponent (L−M) channel, and (c) the second colour opponent (L+M−S) channel, under the assumption of optimum efficiency. The calculations were made by weighting the spectral sensitivities of the L, M, and S receptors as appropriate for a particular chromaticity, and performing principal components analysis to determine the weightings given to the three channels to achieve optimally efficient transmission of information. The spectral sensitivities of the photoreceptors were calculated from the equations given by Hunt (1991). Each receptor was weighted according to the density of cone types in the retina using the factors given in Hunt's model.

The luminance and colour difference channels have no direct parallels in the physiology of the visual system. Both the magnocellular and parvocellular pathways presumably carry information about luminance. The magnocellular pathway differs from the parvo, however, in that it is not supposed to carry information about colour differences. If the 'magnocellular' pathways were impaired, as in some people with dyslexia, one might suppose that this impairment would affect the efficiency of transmission of luminance information. A similar loss of efficiency might occur in people complaining of glare. Improvements in signal transmission would then result when the information on the luminance channel was reduced and that on the colour difference channels increased. This is achieved with optimal efficiency when the receptor sensitivities are those that would obtain with blue illuminants. We saw in the previous chapter that many (but not all) of the children with reading difficulties reported that a bluish hue reduced the perceptual distortion of text (Fig. 9.5(h)).

10.3 Synthesis

At the end of the previous chapter we proposed a unified theory for the effectiveness of coloured glasses in dyslexia, migraine, and photosensitive epilepsy. In essence, it was proposed that cortical hyperexcitability was responsible for perceptual distortions and for triggering migraine and epilepsy. The characteristics of the hyperexcitability appeared to implicate the magnocellular more than the parvocellular pathways. The tints were supposed to redistribute the patterning of nervous activity in cortical networks so as to avoid areas of hyperexcitability. In this chapter we have seen that the hyperexcitability might be further enhanced by damage to visual pathways during migraine attacks and that the tints may restore efficient signal transmission over pathways that have been damaged. We have also seen that the visual stimuli that give rise to discomfort are those that may place an excessive computational demand upon the processes by which the visual scene is grouped. We are left with the picture of a slightly compromised visual system that malfunctions when computational demand is excessive.

10.4 Caveat

The ideas in this chapter are speculations and not to be taken too seriously. As Mark Twain once observed, 'There is something wonderful about science: one gets such wholesale return of conjecture from so trifling an investment of fact'.

Appendix: Techniques for treatment

Various techniques for treating visual discomfort are summarized.

In the preceding chapters, temporal and spatial characteristics of visual stimulation have been identified as responsible for visual discomfort. Pulsation of light that is too rapid to see as flicker can induce eye-strain and headaches, and lower frequency flicker can cause epileptic seizures as well. Spatially repetitive patterns, such as stripes, can have effects similar to those of flicker. In this chapter we review techniques for avoiding these unfortunate effects. The purpose is not to provide a complete review, but to refer the reader to those chapters where the issue is discussed in detail.

A.1 Prevention of photosensitive seizures

Patients with photosensitive epilepsy are at risk of seizures when exposed to flickering light, such as discotheque strobes and sunlight passing through road-side trees. Simply closing the eyes is no protection. The light diffuses through the eyelids, increasing the area of retina exposed, which can exacerbate the effects. When exposed to flicker, patients should not close the eyes but should cover one eye with the palm of a hand (Jeavons and Harding 1975). The effects of flicker are usually greatly reduced when the stimulation is monocular (see Section 2.2.3).

Flicker from television is one of the principle causes of seizures in patients with photosensitive epilepsy. Patients should sit at a distance of at least 2 m from the television (more than three times the width of the screen). If they have to go near the screen they should cover one eye with the palm of a hand. In Chapter 7 we gave details of polarized glasses that provide a selective and cosmetic way of preventing light from the television reaching one eye. Some of the new television technologies (100 Hz television, liquid crystal screens) will be beneficial in reducing seizures.

As we saw in Chapter 8, the design of wallpaper and furnishings can be a problem if it provides a repetitive pattern.

There is the possibility that coloured glasses may help prevent seizures in certain cases, as described in Chapter 9. Although treatment with precision tints is available in certain optometric practices, it is advisable for patients with photosensitive epilepsy to be assessed for precision tints in a hospital, if possible with concurrent EEG monitoring. This will necessitate a liaison between optometrists and encephalographers.

Summary

- Cover one eye when exposed to flicker.

- Watch television from at least 2 m or obtain a liquid crystal television.

- Avoid striped furnishings and clothing.

A.2 Headaches and eye-strain from lighting

In Chapter 6 various techniques for avoiding the unpleasant effects of fluorescent lighting were described. People who suffer headaches and eye-strain from fluorescent lighting may find the following steps helpful:

(1) try and sit as near a window as possible (avoiding direct sunlight), so that the daylight reduces the depth of modulation of the flicker;

(2) substitute a tungsten – halogen uplighter for the fluorescent lamps in their immediate vicinity; or

(3) substitute warm white lamps which have a lower modulation;

(4) try and arrange for high-frequency electronic circuitry at the next lighting refit;

(5) obtain glasses that have been tinted in such a way that they reduce the amount of pulsating light reaching the eyes.

A tint suitable for reducing pulsation is described in Chapter 6.[1] It reduces the pulsation from the widely used halophosphate lamps (white, warm white, cool white) but not from triphosphor lamps (Colour 84, Polylux etc.). The tint has been shown to reduce headaches in school children in a small scale but double-blind study. There are large individual differences in the tolerance to coloured glasses, and some people find the colour unpleasantly strong. It is therefore essential to try out a demonstration pair before purchase.

Summary

- Avoid or 'dilute' the light from fluorescent lamps.

- Consider glasses with a tint that reduces the flicker.

---

[1] The *Comfort 41*® tint is manufactured by Cambridge Optical Group, Bar Hill, Cambridge, and is obtainable from high street optometrists.

A.3 Headaches, eye-strain, and seizures from reading

Repetitive patterns can also be uncomfortable to look at, inducing eye-strain, headaches, and even seizures. Chapter 5 showed that printed text resembles a pattern of stripes. Eye-strain and headaches and seizures can sometimes be prevented by a simple mask[1] that darkens and blurs the unnecessary lines.

In Chapter 9 we described the use of tinted glasses and overlays in reducing perceptual distortion of text. Tinting using Irlen's techniques is available privately from the Irlen Institute[2]. Tinting using the Intuitive Colorimeter[3] is available at certain optometric practices in Britain, and elsewhere[4].

Coloured plastic sheets placed upon a page of text (overlays),[5] offer an inexpensive alternative to tinted glasses. Indeed the British College of Optometrists recommend that before children receive tinted lenses they should have used overlays for a trial period. This method of treatment has received little research, but it appears that the colour needs to be selected from a large range of filters, using appropriate methods of presentation. The colours that are found to be beneficial when using overlays are *hardly ever* the same as those that are beneficial in glasses.

The subject should compare each of the overlays in turn to decide whether the filter results in an improvement, a deterioration, or has no effect. When the filters that improve perception have a colour complementary to the colour of those that make matters worse, one can have greater confidence that colour *per se* is responsible for the effects. When several overlays improve perception, they should be compared side by side, two at a time, under a variety of lighting conditions. The best one can then be selected by a process of elimination.

If the subject benefits from the use of a coloured overlay, this will be revealed in a change in attitude to reading, a willingness to read for longer, and possibly also an improvement in reading fluency and a reduction in headaches. Subjects who benefit in this way from the use of an overlay, may find appropriately coloured spectacles of greater convenience and sometimes of greater benefit, presumably due to the greater precision of colour choice.

---

[1] The *Cambridge Easy Reader* is manufactured by Engineering and Design Plastics, Cherry Hinton, Cambridge, and is obtainable by post.

[2] The Irlen Institute has many branches in the USA and throughout the world, including one in London.

[3] The *Intuitive Colorimeter* is manufactured by Cerium Optical Group Ltd, Tenterden, Kent.

[4] For a list of optometrists that have the Intuitive Colorimeter, contact the Institute of Optometry in London.

[5] The Institute of Optometry in London supply 'Intuitive Overlays'. Ten colours are available in an Assessment Pack, and individual colours can also be obtained separately.

Summary

- Choose book editions with large widely spaced text, where possible.

- Try masking the text above and below, leaving three lines visible for reading.

- Try a range of coloured overlays, selecting the most comfortable.

- If the overlays are helpful, try glasses with precision tints.

A.4 Colour in therapy: a caveat

We saw in Chapter 6 that certain people are sensitive to the rapid pulsation of light from fluorescent lamps. The pulsation affects the control of eye movements and increases headaches. It can be removed using new electronic circuitry, with a consequent reduction in headaches among office workers. The pulsation can also be reduced by wearing spectacles that selectively absorb light with wavelengths less than 550 nm, and these have been shown to reduce migraine headaches among school children. The reduction of headaches is easy to understand on a physical basis. The spectacles reduce the depth of modulation of the light by about 30 per cent. This may seem a small reduction, but it is sufficient to change the visibility of lower frequency flicker by a large amount. Moreover modulation from fluorescent lamps is usually reduced by 'dilution' with daylight. The 30 per cent contribution from the glasses may therefore be sufficient to remove the physiological consequences of the pulsation.

The colours of tints that reduce pulsation from fluorescent lamps exacerbate pattern glare in some people. The lens that reduces the flicker from fluorescent lamps (see Section 6.10) has a reddish hue and, as we have seen, pattern glare is most commonly reduced by colours *complementary* to red. In general, tints that absorb wavelengths less than 550 nm have colours that lie in the right-hand half of the UCS diagram. This area is opposite the area most frequently chosen to reduce pattern glare from text (see Fig. 9.5(h)).

If the above analysis is correct, and it is too soon to be sure, the choice of a tint colour that is likely to be beneficial will be determined by the relative contribution of two factors: susceptibility to fluorescent lighting and susceptibility to pattern glare. The choice of examination procedure needs to be determined by the clinical history. If the history implicates an aversion to fluorescent lighting, it is not sufficient to use a colorimeter with stable illumination to measure a comfortable tint. The colorimeter provides an estimate of the role of colour in reducing pattern glare, but if susceptibility to flicker is part of the clinical problem, the setting needs to be confirmed using trial lenses under conditions of fluorescent lighting that approximate those the patient normally experiences.

Summary

- An individual's sensitivity to flicker and to pattern may require incompatible colours. Both sources of discomfort need to be considered together.

References

Anthony, M. and Lance, J.W. (1975). The role of serotonin in migraine. In: *Modern topics in migraine* (ed. J. Pearce), pp. 107–23. Heinemann, London.

Arundale, K. (1978). An investigation into the variation of human contrast sensitivity with age and ocular pathology. *British Journal of Ophthalmology*, **62**, 213–15.

Barbur, J. and Ruddock, K.H. (1980). Spatial characteristics of movement detection mechanisms in human vision. I Achromatic vision. *Biological Cybernetics*, **37**, 77–92.

Baron, R.A., Rea, M.S., and Daniels, S.G. (1992). Effects of indoor lighting (illuminance and spectral distribution) on the performance of cognitive tasks and interpersonal behaviors: the potential mediating role of positive affect. *Motivation and Emotion*, **16**(1), 1–33.

Beazley, R.D., Illingworth, D.J., John, A., and Green, D.V. (1980). Contrast sensitivity in children and adults. *British Journal of Ophthalmology*, **64**, 863–6.

Benham, C.E. (1894). The artificial spectrum top. *Nature*, **51**, 200.

Berman, N.J., Douglas R.J., and Martin, K.A.C. (1992) GABA-mediated inhibition in the neural networks of visual-cortex. *Progress in Brain Research*, **90**, 443–76.

Berman, S.M., Greenhouse, D.S., Bailey, I.L., Clear, R.D., and Raasch, T.W. (1991). Human electroretinogram responses to video displays, fluorescent lighting, and other high frequency sources. *Optometry and Vision Science*, **68**(8), 645–62.

Bickford, R.G., Daly, D., and Keith, H.M. (1953). Convulsive effects of light stimulation in children. *American Journal of Diseases of Children*, **86**, 170–83.

Bidwell, S. (1896). On subjective colour phenomena attending sudden changes in illumination. *Proceedings of the Royal Society*, **60**, 368–77.

Binnie, C.D., Darby, C.E., and Wilkins, A.J. (1979*a*). Pattern-sensitivity: The role of movement. In *Proceedings of the second European congress of electroencephalography and clinical neurophysiology* (ed. H. Lechner and A. Avanibar); pp. 650–5. Elsevier, North Holland.

Binnie, C.D., de Korte, R.A., and Wisman, T. (1979*b*). Fluorescent lighting and epilepsy. *Epilepsia*, **20**, 725–7.

Binnie, C.D., Wilkins, A.J., and de Korte, R.A. (1981). Interhemispheric differences in photosensitivity: II. Intermittent photic stimulation. *Electroencephalography and Clinical Neurophysiology*, **52**, 469–72.

Binnie, C.D., Estevez, O., Kasteleijn-Nolst Trenité, D.G.A., and Peters, A. (1984). Colour and photosensitive epilepsy. *Electroencephalography and Clinical Neurophysiology*, **58**, 387–91.

Binnie, C.D., Findlay, J., and Wilkins, A.J. (1985). Mechanisms of epileptogenesis in photosensitive epilepsy implied by the effects of moving patterns. *Electroencephalography and Clinical Neurophysiology*, **61**, 1–6.

Blau, J.N. and Drummond, M.F. (1991). *Migraine*. Office of Health Economics, London.

Blakemore, C. and Campbell, F.W. (1969). On the existence in the human visual system of neurones selectively sensitive to the orientation and size of retinal images. *Journal of Physiology (London)*, **203**, 237–60.

Blumhardt, L.D., Barrett, G., Halliday, A.M., and Kriss, A. (1978). The effect of experimental 'scotomata' on the ipsilateral and contralateral responses to pattern-reversal in one half-field. *Electroencephalography and Clinical Neurophysiology*, **45**, 376–92.

Bodis-Wollner, I. and Diamond, S.P. (1973). A method of testing and evaluating blurred vision in cerebral lesions. *Transactions of the American Neurological Association*, **98**, 57–60.

Boer, M.O. den, Villalón, C.M., Heiligers, J.P.C., Humphrey, P.P.A., and Saxena, P.R. (1991). Role of 5-HT[1]-like receptors in the reduction of porcine cranial arteriovenous anastomotic shunting by sumatriptan. *British Journal of Pharmacology*, **102**, 323–30.

Botnton, R.M. and Nagy, A.L. (1982). La Jolla analytic colorimeter. *Journal of the Optical Society of America* **72**, 666–7.

Brewster, Sir D. (1832). On the undulations excited in the retina by the action of luminous points and lines. *London and Edinburgh Philosophical Magazine and Journal of Science*, **1**, 169–74.

Brindley, G.S. (1962). Beats produced by simultaneous stimulation of the human eye with intermittent light and intermittent or alternating electric current. *Journal of Physiology (London)*, **164**, 157–67.

Brundrett, G.W. (1974). Human sensitivity to flicker. *Lighting Research and Technology*, **6**(3), 127–43.

Buchsbaum, G. (1987). Color signal coding: color vision and color television. *Color Research and Application*, **12**(5), 266–9.

Buchsbaum, G. and Gottschalk, A. (1983). Trichromacy, opponent colour coding and optimum colour information transmission in the retina. *Proceedings of the Royal Society of London B*, **220**, 89–113.

Burnham, R.W. (1952). A colorimeter for research in colour perception. *American Journal of Psychology*, **65**, 603–8.

Campbell, F.W. and Maffei, L. (1974). Contrast and spatial frequency. *Scientific American*, **231**(5), 106–14.

Campbell, F.W. and Robson, J.G. (1968). Application of Fourier analysis to the visibility of gratings. *Journal of Physiology*, **197**, 551–66.

Carterette, E.C. and Symmes, D. (1952). Colour as an experimental variable in photic stimulation. *Electroencephalography and Clinical Neurophysiology*, **4**, 289–96.

Chatrian, G.E., Lettich, E., Miller, L.H., and Green, J.R. (1970). Pattern-sensitive epilepsy. Part 1. An electroencephalographic study of its mechanisms. *Epilepsia*, **15**, 125–49.

Chen, T.C. and Leviton, A. (1990). Asthma and eczema in children born to women with migraine. *Archives of Neurology*, **47**(11), 1227–30.

Chronicle, E.P. and Wilkins, A.J. (1991). Colour and visual discomfort in migraineurs. *Lancet*, **338**, 890.

Clark, B.A.J. (1969). Colour in sunglass lenses. *American Journal of Optometry and Archives of the American Academy of Optometry*, **46**, 825–40.

Cohen, J. and Gordon, D.A. (1949). The Prévost-Fechner-Benham subjective colours. *Psychological Bulletin*, **46**, 2.

Collins, R.E.C. (1969). A new escalator injury. *Lancet*, **i**, 1268.

Corbett, J.M. and White, T.A. (1976). Visibility of flicker in television pictures, *Nature*, **261**, 689–90.

Courjon, J. (1955). La protection des épileptiques photogéniques par des verres filtrant la partie rouge du spectre. *Revue d'oto-neuro-ophtalmologie*, **27**, 462–3.

Dainoff, M.J. (1982). Occupational stress factors in visual display terminal (VDT) operation: A review of empirical research. *Behaviour and Information Technology*, **1**(2), 141–76.

Darby, C.E., Wilkins, A.J., Binnie, C.D., and de Korte, R.A. (1980). Routine testing for pattern sensitivity. *Journal of Electrophysiological Technology*, **6**, 202–10.

Darby, C.E., Park, D.M., and Wilkins, A.J. (1986). EEG characteristics of epileptic pattern sensitivity and their relation to the nature of pattern stimulation and the effects of sodium valproate. *Electroencephalography and Clinical Neurophysiology*, **63**, 517–25.

De Lange, H. (1952). Experiments on flicker and some calculations on an electrical analogue of the foveal systems. *Physica*, **18** (11), 935–50.

Derefeldt, G., Lennerstrand, G., and Lundh, B. (1979). Age variations in normal human contrast sensitivity. *Acta Ophthalmologica (Kjøbenhavn)*, **57**, 679–90.

Derrico, J.B. and Buchsbaum, G. (1991). A computational model of spatiochromatic image coding in early vision. *Journal of Visual Communication and Image Representation*, **2**(1), 31–8.

Drasdo, N. (1977). The neural representation of visual space. *Nature (London)*, **266**, 554–6.

Evans, B.J.W. and Drasdo, N. (1990). Review of ophthalmic factors in dyslexia. *Ophthalmic and Physiological Optics*, **10**, 200–9.

Evans, B.J.W. and Drasdo, N. (1991). Tinted lenses and related therapies for learning difficulties – a review. *Ophthalmic and Physiological Optics*, **11**, 206–17.

Evans, J. (1987). Women, men, VDU work and health: A questionnaire survey of British VDU operators. *Work and Stress*, **1**(3), 271–83.

Eysel, U.T. and Burandt, U. (1984). Fluorescent tube light evokes flicker responses in visual neurones. *Vision Research*, **24**, 943–8.

Ferster D. (1986). Orientation selectivity of synaptic potentials in neurons of cat primary visual cortex. *Journal of Neuroscience*, **6** (5), 1284–301.

Findlay, J.M. (1982). Global processing for saccadic eye movements. *Vision Research*, **22**, 1033–45.

Fox, P.T. and Raichle, M.E. (1984). Stimulus rate dependence of regional cerebral blood flow in human striate cortex, demonstrated by position emission tomography. *Journal of Neurophysiology*, **51** (5), 1109–20.

Georgeson, M.A. (1976). Psychophysical hallucinations of orientation and spatial frequency. *Perception*, **5**, 99–111.

Georgeson, M.A. (1980). The perceived spatial frequency, contrast and orientation of illusory gratings. *Perception*, **9**, 695–712.

Gilbert, C.D. and Wiesel, T.N. (1983). Clustered intrinsic connections in cat visual cortex. *Journal of Neuroscience*. 3, 1116–33.

Gilbert, C.D. and Wiesel, T.N. (1989). Columnar specificity of intrinsic horizontal and corticocortical connections in cat visual cortex. *Journal of Neuroscience*, 9, 2432–42.

Gloor, P. (1986). Migraine and regional cerebral upflow. *Trends in Neurosciences*, 9, 21.

Goldensohn, E.S. (1976). Paroxysmal and other features of the electroencephalogram in migraine. *Research and Clinical Studies in Headache*, 4, 118–28.

Golla, F.L. and Winter, A.L. (1959). Analysis of cerebral responses to flicker in patients complaining of episodic headache. *Electroencephalography and Clinical Neurophysiology*, 11, 539–49.

Good, P.A., Taylor, R.H., and Mortimer, M.J. (1991). The use of tinted glasses in childhood migraine. *Headache*, 31, 533–6.

Grounds, A.R., Holliday, I.E., and Ruddock, K.H. (1983). Two spatio-temporal filters in human vision. II Selective modification in amblyopia, albinism and hemianopia. *Biological Cybernetics*, 47, 191–201.

Harwood, K. and Foley, P. (1987). Temporal resolution: an insight into the video display terminal (VDT) 'problem.' *Human Factors*, 29(4), 447–52.

Hata, Y., Tsumoto, T., Sato, H., Hagihara, H. *et al.* (1988). Inhibition contributes to orientation selectivity in visual cortex of cat. *Nature* 335 (6193), 815–17.

Hazell, J. and Wilkins, A.J. (1990). A contribution of fluorescent lighting to agoraphobia. *Psychological Medicine*, 20, 591–6.

Hering, R. and Kuritzky, A. (1992). Sodium valproate in the phrophylactic treatment of migraine: a double-blind study versus placebo. *Cephalagia*, 12, 81–4.

Hess, R.F. and Howell, E.R. (1977). The threshold contrast sensitivity function in strasbismic amblyopia: evidence for a two-type classification. *Vision Research*, 17, 1049–55.

Heyck, H. (1969). Pathogenesis of migraine. *Research and Clinical Studies in Headache* 2. Ed. A. Friedman. Karger, Basel, pp. 1–28.

Heyhoe, M. and Wenderoth, P. (1991). Adaptation mechanisms in colour and brightness. In *From pigments to perception* (ed. A. Valberg and B.B. Lee), pp. 353–67. Plenum Press, New York.

Holliday, I.E. and Ruddock, K.H. (1983). Two spatio-temporal filters in human vision. I Temporal and spatial frequency response characteristics. *Biological Cybernetics*, 47, 173–90.

Horton, J.C. and Hubel, D.H. (1981). A regular patchy distribution of cytochrome-oxidase staining in primary visual cortex of the macaque monkey. *Nature*, 292, 762–4.

Howarth, P.A. and Istance, H.O. (1985). The association between visual discomfort and the use of visual display units. *Behaviour and Information Technology*, 4(2), 131–49.

Hubel, D.H. (1988). *Eye, brain and vision*. W.H. Freeman, New York.

Humphrey, A.L. and Hendrickson A.E. (1983). Background and stimulus-induced patterns of high metabolic activity in the visual cortex (area 17) of the squirrel and macaque monkey. *Journal of Neuroscience*, 3 (2), 345–58.

Hunt, R.W.G. (1987). *Measuring colour*. Ellis Horwood, Chichester.

Hunt, R.W.G. (1991). *Measuring colour*. (2nd edn). Ellis Horwood, Chichester.

Irlen, H. (1983). *Successful treatment of learning disabilities*. Unpublished paper presented at First Annual Convention of American Psychological Association, Annheim, Ca.

Irlen H. (1991). *Reading by the colors: overcoming dyslexia and other reading disabilities through the Irlen method*. Avery Publishing Group, New York.

Ives, J.R., Wilkins, A., Jones, M., Andermann, F., and Woods, J. (1976). Twenty-seven days in the life of an epileptic patient. *Biotelemetry*, **3**, 177–80.

Jeavons, P.M. and Harding, G.F.A. (1975). *Photosensitive epilepsy: a review of the literature and a study of 460 patients*. Heinemann, London.

Jonkman, E.J. and Lelieveld, M.H. (1981). EEG computer analysis in patients with migraine. *Electroencephalography and Clinical Neurophysiology*, **52**, 652–5.

Kelly, D.H. (1972). Flicker. In *Handbook of Sensory Physiology*, Vol. 7, No. 4 (ed. D. Jameson and L.M. Hurvich), pp. 273–302. Springer-Verlag, New York.

Kennedy, A. and Murray, W.S. (1991). The effects of flicker on eye movement control. *Quarterly Journal of Experimental Psychology*, **43A**(1), 79–99.

Khalil, N. (1991). *Investigations of visual function in migraine by visual evoked potentials and visual psychophysical tests*. Unpublished PhD Thesis, University of London.

Land, E.H. (1977). The retinex theory of color vision. *Scientific American*, **237**, 108–28.

Laubli, Th., Hunting, W., and Grandjean, E. (1983). Visual impairments in VDU operators related to environmental conditions. In *Ergonomic aspects of visual display terminals* (ed. E. Grandjean and E. Vigliani), Taylor and Francis, London.

Lauritzen, M., Jorgensen, M.B., Diemer, N.H., Gjedde, A., and Hansen, A.J. (1982). Persistent oligemia of rat cerebral cortex in the wake of spreading depression. *Annals of Neurology*, **12**, 469–74.

Leão, A.A.P. (1944). Spreading depression of activity in the cerebral cortex. *Journal of Neurophysiology*, **7**, 359–90.

Lehtonen, J. (1974). Visual evoked cortical potentials for single flashes and flickering light in migraine. *Headache*, **14**, 1–12.

Liberman, J. (1986). The effect of syntonic (colored light) stimulation on certain visual and cognitive functions. *Journal of Optometric Vision Development*, **17**, 1–11.

Livingston, S. (1952). Comments on a study of light-induced epilepsy in children. *American Journal of Diseases of Children*, **83**, 409.

Livingston, S. (1972). *Comprehensive management of epilepsy in infancy, childhood and adolescence*. CC Thomas, Springfield, Il.

Livingstone, M.S. and Hubel, D.H. (1987). Psychophysical evidence for separate channels for the perception of form, colour, movement, and depth. *Journal of Neuroscience*, **7**(11), 3416–68.

Livingstone, M.S. and Hubel, D. (1988). Segregation of form, color, movement, and depth: anatomy physiology and perception. *Science*, **240**, 740–9.

Livingstone, M.S., Rosen, G.D., Drislane, F.W., and Galaburda, A.M. (1991).

Physiological and anatomical evidence for a magnocellular defect in developmental dyslexia. *Proceedings of the National Academy of Sciences of the United States of America*, **88**, 7943–7.

Lovegrove, W., Martin, F., and Slaghuis, W. (1986). A theoretical and experimental case for a residual deficit in specific reading disability. *Cognitive Neuropsychology*, **3**, 225–67.

Mackay, D. (1961). Interactive processes in visual perception. In *Sensory communication* (ed. W.A. Rosenblith), pp. 339–55. J. Wiley, London.

Maclachlan, A., Yale, S., and Wilkins, A.J. (1993). Open trials of precision ophthalmic tinting: 1-year follow-up of 55 patients. *Opthalmic and Physiological Optics*, **13**, 175–8.

Marcus, D.A. and Soso, M.J. (1989). Migraine and stripe-induced discomfort. *Archives of Neurology*, **46**, 1129–32.

Marr, D.C. (1982). *Vision*. W.H. Freeman & Co., San Francisco.

Marshall, C., Walker, A.E., and Livingston, S. (1953). Photogenic epilepsy: parameters of activation. *Archives of Neurology*, **69**, 760–5.

Martin, K.A.C. (1992). Parallel pathways converge. *Current Biology*, **2** (10), 555–7.

Matin, E., Clymer, A., and Matin, L. (1972). Metacontrast and saccadic suppression. *Science*, **178**, 179–82.

McKinlay, A.F., Whillock, M.J., and Meulemans, C.C.E. (1989). *Ultraviolet radiation and blue-light emissions from spotlights incorporating tungsten halogen lamps*, National Radiation Protection Board technical report 228. HMSO London.

Meares, O. (1980). Figure/background, brightness/contrast and reading disabilities. *Visible Language*, **14**, 13–29.

Mehr, E.B. (1969). The typoscope by Charles Prentice. *American Journal of Optometry*, **46**, 885–7.

Meldrum, B.S. and Wilkins, A.J. (1984). Photosensitive epilepsy in man and the baboon: integration of pharmacological and psychophysical evidence. In *Electrophysiology of epilepsy* (ed. P.A. Schwartzkroin and H.V. Wheal), pp. 51–77. Academic Press, London.

Menacker, S.J., Breton, M.L., Radcliffe, J., and Gole, G.A. (1993). Do tinted lenses improve the reading performance of dyslexic children? *Archives of Ophthalmology*, **111**, 213–18.

Milner, P.M. (1958). Note on a possible correspondence between the scotomas of migraine and spreading depression of Leão. *Electroencephalography and Clinical Neurophysiology*, **10**, 705.

Mishkin, M. and Ungerleider, L.G. (1983). Object vision and spatial vision: two cortical pathways. *Trends in Neurosciences*, **6** (10), 414–17.

Moorhead, I.R. (1985). Human colour vision and natural images. In *Colour in information technology and information displays*, Institute of Electronic and Radio Engineers Publication Number 61, p. 21. Alderman, Ipswich.

Morley, S. and Hunter, M. (1983). Temporal artery pulse amplitude wave shapes in migraineurs: a methodological investigation. *Journal of Psychosomatic Research*, **27**(6), 485–92.

Morrone, M.C., Burr, D.C., and Maffei, L. (1982). Functional implications of cross-orientation inhibition of cortical visual cells. I Neurophysiological evidence. *Proceedings of the Royal Society of London*, **B**, 216, 335–54.

Movshon, J.A., Thompson, I.D., and Tolhurst, D.J. (1978). Spatial and temporal contrast sensitivity of neurones in areas 17 and 18 of the cat visual cortex. *Journal of Physiology (London)*, **283**, 101–20.

Neary, C. and Wilkins, A.J. (1989). Effects of phosphor persistence on perception and the control of eye movements. *Perception*, **18**, 257–64.

Newmark, M.E. and Penry, J.K. (1979). *Photosensitivity and epilepsy: a review.* Raven Press, New York.

Njemanze, P.C., Gomez, C.R., and Horenstein, S. (1992). Cerebral lateralization and colour perception: a transcranial doppler study. *Cortex*, **28**, 69–75.

Nulty, D., Wilkins, A.J., and Williams, J.M. (1987). Mood, pattern sensitivity and headache: a longitudinal study. *Psychological Medicine*, **17**, 705–13.

Nyrke, T. and Lang, A.H. (1982). Spectral analysis of visual potentials evoked by sine wave modulated light in migraine. *Electroencephalography and Clinical Neurophysiology*, **53**, 436–42.

O'Connor, P.D., Sofo, F., Kendall, L.S., and Olesen, G. (1990). Reading disabilities and the effects of coloured filters. *Journal of Learning Disabilities*, **23**(10), 597–603.

O'Regan, K. (in press). Eye movements and reading. In *Eye Movements and their role in visual and cognitive processes*. Vol 4 of *Reviews of Oculomotor Research* (ed. E. Knowles). Elsevier, London.

Olesen, J. (1987). The ischemic hypotheses of migraine. *Archives of Neurology*, **44**, 321–2.

Olesen, J. (ed.) (1988). Classification and diagnostic criteria for headache disorders, cranial neuralgias and facial pain. *Cephalagia*, **8**, Supplement 7.

Ottes, F.P., van Gisbergen, J.A.M., and Eggermont, J.J. (1984). Metrics of saccadic responses to double stimuli: two different modes. *Vision Research*, **24**, 1169–79.

Plant, G.T., Zimmern, R.L., and Durden, K. (1983). Transient visually evoked potentials to the pattern reversal and onset of sinusoidal gratings. *Electroencephalography and Clinical Neurophysiology*, **56**, 147–58.

Poulton, E.C. (1959). Effects of printing types and formats on the comprehension of scientific journals. *Nature*, **184**, 1824–5.

Poulton, E.C. (1960). A note on printing to make comprehension easier. *Ergonomics*, **3**(3), 245–8.

Poulton, E.C. (1965). Letter differentiation and rate of comprehension in reading. *Journal of Applied Psychology*, **49**(5), 358–62.

Poulton, E.C. (1979). Models for biases in judging sensory magnitude. *Psychological Bulletin*, **86**, 777–803.

Purkinje, J. (1823). *Beobachtungen and Versuche zur Physiologie der Sinne. Beiträge zur Kenntnis des Sehens in subjectiver Hinsicht Erstes Bändchen.* Calve'scehn Buchhandlung, Prague.

Regan, D., Silver, R., and Murray, T.J. (1977). Visual acuity and contrast sensitivity in multiple sclerosis: hidden visual loss. *Brain*, **100**, 563–70.

Reilly, E.L. and Peters, J.F. (1973). Relationship of some varieties of electroencephalographic photosensitivity to clinical convulsive disorders. *Neurology (Minneapolis)*, **23**, 1050–7.

Rey, P. and Rey, J.P. (1963). Les effects comparés de deux éclairage fluorescents sur une tache visuelle et des tests de 'fatigue'. *Ergonomics*, **6**, 393–401.

Reynolds, L. (1979). Progress in documentation. Legibility studies: their relevance to present-day documentation methods. *Journal of Documentation*, **35**, 307–40.

Richards, W. (1971). The fortification illusions of migraine. *Scientific American*, **224**, 89–96.

Robson, J.G. and Graham, N. (1981). Probability summation and regional variation in contrast sensitivity across the visual field. *Vision Research*, **21**, 409–18.

Rooney, J.C. and Williams, H.E. (1971). The relationship between proved viral bronchiolitis and subsequent wheezing. *Journal of Pediatrics*, **79**(5), 744–7.

Rosner, J. and Rosner, J. (1987). The Irlen treatment: a review of the literature. *Optician*, **25**, September, 26–33.

Saint-John, L.M. and White, M.A. (1988). The effect of coloured transparencies on the reading performance of reading-disabled children. *Australian Journal of Psychology*, **40**(4), 403–11.

Selby, G. and Lance, J.W. (1960). Observations on 500 cases of migraine and allied vascular headache. *Journal of Neurology, Neurosurgery and Psychiatry*, **23**, 23–32.

Sillito, A.M. (1979). Inhibitory mechanisms influencing complex cell orientation selectivity and their modification at high resting discharge levels. *Journal of Physiology (London)*, **289**, 33–53.

Sjörstrand, J. and Frisen, L. (1977). Contrast sensitivity in macular disease. *Acta Ophalmologica (Kjøbenhavn)*, **55**, 507–14.

Skyhoj-Olsen, T. and Lassen, N.A. (1989). Blood flow and vascular activity during attacks of classical migraine. Limitations of intra arterial techniques. *Headache*, **29**, 15–20.

Sly, P.D. and Hibbert, M.E. (1989). Childhood asthma following hospitalization with acute viral bronchiolitis in infancy. *Pediatric Pulmonology*, **7**(3), 153–8.

Smith, A.P., Tyrrell, D.A.J., Barrow, G., Higgings, P.G., Bull, S., Trickett, S., and Wilkins, A.J. (1992). The common cold, pattern sensitivity and contrast sensitivity. *Psychological Medicine*, **22**, 487–94.

Soso, M.J., Lettich, E., and Belgum, J.H. (1980*a*). Case report: responses to stripe width changes and to complex gratings of a patient with pattern-sensitive epilepsy. *Electroencephalography and Clinical Neurophysiology*, **48**, 98–101.

Soso, M.J., Lettich, E., and Belgum, J.H. (1980*b*). Pattern-sensitive epilepsy I: A demonstration of spatial frequency selective epileptic response to gratings. *Epilepsia*, **21**, 301–12.

Soso, M.J., Lettich, E., and Belgum, J.H. (1980*c*). Pattern-sensitive epilepsy II: Effects of pattern orientation and hemifield stimulation. *Epilepsia*, **21**, 313–23.

Spekreijse, H., Estevez, O., and Reits, D. (1977). Visual evoked potentials and the physiological analysis of visual processes in man. In *Visual evoked potentials in man: new developments* (ed. J.E. Desmedt), pp. 16–89. Clarendon Press, Oxford.

Stanley, G. (1991). Glare, scotopic sensitivity and colour therapy. In *Vision and visual dyslexia* (ed. J.F. Stein, Vol. 13 of *Vision and visual Dysfunction* (ed. J. Cronly-Dillon). Macmillan, Basingstoke.

Stefansson, S.B., Darby, C.E., Wilkins, A.J., Binnie, C.D., Malton, A.P., Smith,

A.T., and Stockley, A.V. (1977). Television epilepsy and pattern sensitivity. *British Medical Journal*, **2**, 88–90.

Takahashi, T. and Tsukahara, Y. (1976). Influence of colour on the photoconvulsive response. *Electroencephalography and Clinical Neurophysiology*, **41**, 124–36.

Takahashi, T. and Tsukahara, Y. (1992). Usefulness of blue sunglasses in photosensitive epilepsy. *Epilepsia*, **33**(3), 517–21.

Thompson, W.D. (1985). *Flicker on raster scanned displays as a function of field scan direction*. Unpublished PhD Thesis, City University, London.

Tinker, M.A. (1963). *Legibility of print*. Iowa State University Press, Ames, Iowa.

Tsumoto, T., Eckart, W., and Creutzfeldt, O.D. (1978) Modification of orientation sensitivity of cat visual cortical neurones by removal of GABA-medicated inhibition. *Experimental Brain Research*, **34**, 351–63.

Tyrrell, R., Holland, K., Dennis, D., and Wilkins, A.J. (in press). Coloured overlays, visual discomfort, visual search and classroom reading. *Journal of Research in Reading*.

Van Buskirk, C., Casby, J.U., Passouant, P., and Schwab, R.S. (1959). The effect of different modalities of light on the activation of the EEG. *Electroencephalography and Clinical Neurophysiology*, **11**, 244–5.

Van Harreveld, A. and Stamm, J.S. (1955). Cortical responses to metrazol and sensory stimulation in the rabbit. *Electroencephalography and Clinical Neurophysiology*, **7**, 363–70

Van de Grind, W.A., Grüsser, O.J., and Lunkenheimer, H.U. (1973). Temporal transfer properties of the afferent visual system: psychophysical, neurophysiological and theoretical investigations. In *Handbook of Sensory Physiology*, (ed. R. Jung), Vol. **VII3A**. Springer-Verlag, Berlin.

Vidyasagar, T.R. and Mueller, A. (1994) Function of GABA (A) inhibition in specifying spatial-frequency and orientation selectivities in cat striate cortex. *Experimental Brain Research*, **98** (1), 31–8.

Wade, N.J. (1977). Distortions and disappearance of geometrical patterns. *Perception*, **6**, 407–33.

Watt, R.J. (1991). *Understanding vision*. Academic Press, London.

Watt, R.J. and Morgan, M.J. (1985). A theory of the primitive spatial code in human vision. *Vision Research*, **25**, 1661–74.

Watt, R.J., Bock, J., Thimbleby, H., and Wilkins, A.J. (1990). Visible aspects of text. *Applying visual psychophysics to user interface design*, British Telecom internal report.

Watts, F.N. and Wilkins, A.J. (1989). The role of provocative visual stimuli in agoraphobia. *Psychological Medicine*, **19**, 875–85.

Weston, H.C. (1962). *Sight, light and work*, p.52. Lewis, London.

Wilkins, A.J. (1986). Intermittent illumination from visual display units and fluorescent lighting affects movements of the eyes across text. *Human Factors*, **28**(1), 75–81.

Wilkins, A.J. (1992). Health and efficiency in lighting practice. *Energy*, **18**(2), 123–9.

Wilkins, A.J. (1994). Overlays for classroom and optometric use. *Ophthalmic and Physiological Optics* **14**, 97–9.

Wilkins, A.J. and Clark, C. (1990). Modulation of light from fluorescent lamps. *Lighting Research and Technology*, 22(2), 103–9.

Wilkins, A.J. and Lindsay, J. (1985). Common forms of reflex epilepsy: physiological mechanisms and techniques for treatment. In *Recent advances in epilepsy II* (ed. T.A. Pedley and B.S. Meldrum). Churchill Livingstone, Edinburgh.

Wilkins, A.J. and Neary, C. (1991). Some visual, optometric and perceptual effects of coloured glasses. *Ophthalmic and Physiological Optics*, 11, 163–71.

Wilkins, A.J. and Nimmo-Smith, I. (1984). On the reduction of eye-strain when reading. *Ophthalmic and Physiological Optics*, 4(1), 53–9.

Wilkins, A.J. and Nimmo-Smith, I. (1987). The clarity and comfort of printed text. *Ergonomics*, 30(12), 1705–20.

Wilkins, A.J. and Wilkinson, P. (1991). A tint to reduce eye-strain from fluorescent lighting? Preliminary observations. *Ophthalmic and Physiological Optics*, 11, 172–5.

Wilkins, A.J., Andermann, F., and Ives, J. (1975). Stripes, complex cells and seizures. An attempt to determine the locus and nature of the trigger mechanism in pattern-sensitive epilepsy. *Brain*, 98, 365–80.

Wilkins, A.J., Darby, C.E., and Binnie, C.D. (1979a). Neurophysiological aspects of pattern-sensitive epilepsy. *Brain*, 102, 1–25.

Wilkins, A.J., Darby, C.E., Stefansson, S.F., Jeavons, P.M., and Harding, G.F.A. (1979b). Television epilepsy: the role of pattern. *Electroencephalography and Clinical Neurophysiology*, 47, 163–71.

Wilkins, A.J., Binnie, C.D., and Darby, C.E. (1980). Visually-induced seizures. *Progress in Neurophysiology*, 15, 85–117.

Wilkins, A.J., Binnie, C.D., and Darby, C.E. (1981). Interhemispheric differences in photosensitivity: I. Pattern sensitivity thresholds. *Electroencephalography and Clinical Neurophysiology*, 5, 461–8.

Wilkins, A.J., Nimmo-Smith, I., Tait, A., McManus, C., Della Sala, S., Tilley, A., Arnold, K., Barrie, M., and Scott, S. (1984). A neurological basis for visual discomfort. *Brain*, 107, 989–1017.

Wilkins, A.J., Della Sala, S., Somazzi, L., and Nimmo-Smith, I. (1988). Age-related norms for the Cambridge low contrast gratings, including details concerning their design and use. *Clinical Vision Sciences*, 2(3), 201–12.

Wilkins, A.J., Nimmo-Smith, I., Slater, A., and Bedocs, L. (1989). Fluorescent lighting, headaches and eye-strain. *Lighting Research and Technology*, 21(1), 11–18.

Wilkins, A.J., Milroy, R., Nimmo-Smith, I., Wright, A., Tyrrell, R., Holland, K., Martin, J., Bald, J., Yale, S., Miles, T., and Noakes, T. (1992a). Preliminary observations concerning treatment of visual discomfort and associated perceptual distortion. *Ophthalmic and Physiological Optics*, 12, 257–63.

Wilkins, A.J., Nimmo-Smith, M., and Jansons, J. (1992b). A colorimeter for the intuitive manipulation of hue and saturation, and its application in the study of perceptual distortion. *Ophthalmic and Physiological Optics*, 12, 381–5.

Wilkinson, R.T. and Robinshaw, H.M. (1987). Proof-reading: VDU and paper text compared for speed, accuracy and fatigue. *Behaviour and Information Technology*, 6(2), 125–33.

Williams, M.C., LeCluyse, K., and Rock-Faucheux, A. (1992). Effective interventions for reading disability. *Journal of the Americal Optometric Association*, **63**(6), 411–17.

Winter, A.L. (1987). Neurophysiology and migraine. In *Migraine: clinical, therapeutic conceptual and research aspects* (ed. J.N. Blau). Chapman and Hall, London.

Wolff, H.G. (1963). *Headache and other head pain*. Oxford University Press.

Young, R.S.L., Cole, R.E., Gamble, M., and Rayner, M.D. (1975). Subjective patterns elicited by light flicker. *Vision Research*, **15**, 1291–3.

Zeki, S.M. (1970). Comparision of the cortical degeneration in the visual regions of the temporal lobe of the monkey following section of the anterior commissure and the splenium. *Journal of Comparative Neurology*, **148**, 167–76.

Zeki, S.M. (1978). Functional specialisation in the visual cortex of the rhesus monkey. *Nature (London)*, **274**, 423–8.

Zeki, S.M. (1980). The representation of colours in the cerebral cortex. *Nature (London)*, **284**, 412–18.

Zeki, S.M. (1985). Looking and seeing. In *Scientific basis of clinical neurology* (ed. M. Swash and C. Kennard), pp. 172–87. Churchill Livingstone, Edinburgh.

Index